"We can all agree that our faith should reach into every our lives. But as a former college and professional athlete, I can attest to how difficult it is to inject an authentic walk with Jesus into the arena of physical fitness and competitive sports. Everett offers a unique theological perspective for those who also share these struggles and hope to get themselves on the right path."

—Jason Skaer,
Director of Church Project Network

"Everett Tellez and his wife have a wonderful story of rising up in faith and serving with a passionate purpose. *Faith-Infused Training* highlights the truth that health and fitness empower believers to better serve God and others."

—Betty Okino,
USA Gymnastics Olympic medalist

"*Faith-Infused Training* brings a fresh and unique perspective that challenges us to live every day purposefully with foundational truths. I recommend this book to anyone who seeks to effectively live in their God-given purpose."

—Daryl Jones,
Former MLB player

FAITH-INFUSED

TRAINING

A BIBLICAL PERSPECTIVE OF HEALTH & FITNESS

EVERETT TELLEZ

LUCIDBOOKS

Faith-Infused Training
A Biblical Perspective of Health & Fitness

ISBN-10: 1-63296-234-9
ISBN-13: 978-1-63296-234-8
eISBN-10: 1-63296-235-7
eISBN-13: 978-1-63296-235-5

Special Sales: Most Lucid Books titles are available in special quantity discounts. Custom imprinting or excerpting can also be done to fit special needs. Contact Lucid Books at Info@LucidBooksPublishing.com.

TABLE OF CONTENTS

THIS BOOK IS DEDICATED TO

Mom and Dad,
Steve & Terri Trickel,
Andrew & Kate Howorth

Thanks for always being there for me and my family.
Love, Everett

SPECIAL THANKS

This book could not have been written without the great help and expert tutelage of Dave Edwards, the man behind the manuscript. Dave is in many ways my mentor, but in every way my friend and big brother in Christ. Dave tirelessly serves as the pastor of discipleship at Church Project in The Woodlands, Texas, where I have attended for years. He was the first person I reached out to when this book was just an idea, a dream. Because of his brotherly commitment to me, the goal of getting the message of faith-infused training into the hands and hearts of many has now become an achievement in Christ.

I believe God sent me Dave as an answer to prayer to make that dream come true. I will be indebted to him for as long as I live. His inspiration, his encouragement, and his instruction have made me a stronger believer, a more effective writer, and a more enduring follower of Jesus, all made possible by the amazing grace of God, who used Dave to help me discover the power of scripture in my own testimony.

Dave is an amazing author and dynamic speaker who has served me well. Many can benefit from his gifted writing and speaking. Check him out online at www.daveedwardsspeaks.com.

Also, thanks to Jeremy Ashida, singer, songwriter, and worship pastor at Church Project in Greeley, Colorado. His music was such a huge inspiration and encouragement to me that I included the lyrics to one of his songs in this book. Those lyrics served as great background music during my workouts at the gym and in times of reflection while writing. Download *Church Project Volume 1* on your favorite music app today, and you'll know exactly what I'm talking about.

FOREWORD

I wish I had known Everett when I was in school. I might have excelled in my pursuit of fitness. I'm not an athlete. My memories of playing sports were traumatizing. I'm not too proud to tell you that I once struck out in kickball. Who does that? I mean, how bad do you have to be to miss that big giant red ball three times in a row? After a while I got used to hearing, "Edwards, you're out!"

Do you know what's worse than striking out in kickball? Striking out in T-ball. In T-ball, the ball is not even in motion, and there I was at home plate, swinging away at a motionless ball. Oh, how that ball mocked me.

I spent most of my life hearing all kinds of derogatory comments related to my athletic ability. I remember playing volleyball and serving the ball right into the back of a teammate's head. "Edwards, you're terrible!" Again, the comments—like I needed to be told I was bad.

I reverted to more solitary sports. I lifted weights for a while, but they were so heavy. They say weightlifting is a sport. I disagree. It's picking heavy things up and setting them back down. And why do they call them free weights when you have to pay to use them? I took up running for a short time but soon figured out, "Why should I run when I can drive?"

There's no career for me in athletics in the foreseeable future. However, if I'm to do all God has called me to do, I still need to stay healthy and fit. Following Jesus and bringing expression to the will of God requires a tremendous amount of strength and stamina.

When we survey the landscape of those who walked in the ways of God, they set the standard for us to follow. It's easy to see their journeys weren't for the faint of heart or the physically weak.

It took a level of fitness for God's followers to be fully faithful. Abraham, well into his golden years, climbed Mount Moriah. Moses's assignment made physical fitness a necessity as well. He led millions of people across the desert to the Promised Land. The thought alone is enough to make a professional athlete's heart tremble. The biblical hero and warrior King David fought many battles in his time. Only someone fit could have endured so many confrontations, conflicts, and conquests. Truly, our theology and fitness are connected.

Jesus is the ultimate display of strength. Bearing the physical weight of the cross, which weighed upward of 100 pounds or more, He grabbed hold of one end of the cross beam with two hands, while the rest of the cross was supported by His back and shoulder. While He was nailed to it, He prayed for His enemies. Jesus was no meek, weak, fragile savior. He endured the worst that life had to offer and rose again to give us hope. All the Bible greats needed to be in physical shape. They also needed one more thing—faith.

The road of fitness intersects the way of faith. Faith is not something we add on to what we are already doing. It's a way of life that calls us to unlearn the bad habits we've been living with all these years. It calls for longsuffering reorientation in the resurrection. The ambition that brings about lasting fitness is the ambition infused with faith.

Everett has hit upon the lost ingredient to succeeding in personal fitness. It doesn't include more charts, indexes, or graphs. It's the element of faith. Here in *Faith-Infused Training*, the pages are filled with personal insight. Everett shows us that pursuing fitness with love, grace, humility, righteousness, and holiness is the catalyst of health.

Even today, with my memory seared with the screams and jeers from the sidelines just because I was running the wrong way on the field, I need a voice of encouragement—to keep me focused, to keep me going, to keep me believing, and to keep me pursuing. Every one of us needs someone who can come alongside with words of truth and wisdom to encourage, admonish, and help.

That is what it's like to read *Faith-Infused Training*. Everett writes as a friend, mentor, and encourager. He's personal and transparent about his own life and has lived every single word in this book. I pray you will take the message to heart and infuse your eating habits with faith. Infuse your workout routines with the faith of God. Use Everett's book as a field guide. Mark it up and highlight the passages that speak to you.

No matter what your fitness level is right now, you can be greater, better, stronger, and healthier than you imagined. You are capable of achieving more and accomplishing great things for God. All you need is the hard work of making better choices and, of course, faith.

—Dr. David Edwards, speaker, author *(Life Verse)*
Pastor of Discipleship, Church Project, The Woodlands, Texas

INTRODUCTION

Since becoming a born-again Christian in late 2001, I have sensed a strong call to vocational ministry. I imagine every new believer has that same experience. The joy of salvation produces an excitement in the heart, which sets a fire in our bones to completely transform our lives by giving everything over to God. People quit their jobs, for example, to become missionaries abroad. College students change their majors and enroll in seminary, and musicians leave their rock bands to apply their talents to worship music.

For me, it wasn't so simple. I had no money, no education, and zero criteria. The most I could do was volunteer, as my pastors would tell me, to "serve into ministry." I'd later attend every men's meeting and retreat and all the discipleship seminars and conferences I could find. I also filled out a few internship applications and hung out with 20 or so other guys that felt called, just like me.

Several years later, those guys had all pretty much pursued other options. Some got married and landed big jobs, some realized they lacked compassion and desire, and others prayed about it and God steered them in a different direction. Right around that time is when I decided I should try to make something else happen with my life. Nothing leading to full-time ministry was panning out. Even though I wasn't losing interest, I was quickly losing hope, so much that I began running away from the call to ministry.

That's when a lot of things went south in my life. I turned to many vices that weren't good for my health at all. I got skinny and scrawny during the warm seasons and then bloated and chubby for the holidays, without any idea of how to care for my body. Looking back, I was constantly lying to myself, saying things like this: *You'll never be good enough. You're a hypocrite. You're mediocre, just face it.*

I bought into those lies and let myself tumble down a dark path into an ugly pit. One night while driving drunk, I wrecked a dear friend's car. I think shortly after that, I wrecked his truck. Then, I wrecked my body. After buzzing off a few beers one day, I decided to take my first motorcycle lesson. Minutes into it, I lost control of the bike, crashed into a mailbox, and broke my arm. I spent months in a cast before having surgery, then months more in physical therapy. I had a lot of heart-to-heart conversations with people that year, but the most memorable one was with my doctor at the final visit for my completely healed arm. "You need to start strengthening your body and strengthening that arm," he said. "Eat better. No more smoking. No more heavy drinking."

I took his advice. I joined a gym and started regularly attending Alcoholics Anonymous. It's amazing what a difference it makes to eat healthier and talk to others about your problems. Getting fit and staying sober became huge priorities for me. But even though I had people around me for support, I continued to feel alone and depressed. There were a few significant voids in my life, so I began to fill them with what I thought was best. My life was changing, but regardless of what I did, it was still off. I was still stuck in a dark ugly pit. It had just become more comfortable inside, like I'd found a way to deal with it.

All the steps I was taking toward change simply allowed me access into other people's pits and them into mine. It wasn't so lonely anymore. By the time a year or two went by, I had tunneled through the dark underground of despair and made quite a few friends and acquaintances. I learned to live without the light. Another way of saying that is that I found a way to make darkness appear to be light and settled for that over the light of the world—Jesus. I wore the goodness of God on the outside, but on the inside, I was rotting at the core. My body was changing externally, but underneath all the muscle and tone were polluted lungs, an abused liver, and a hypertensive heart.

That's when I met my future bride, Brittany, who was in a dark pit of her own. God brought us together to remind us that the Christian life isn't meant to be lived underground in despair. He reminded us that we'd been freed by Him from an ungodly and unhealthy lifestyle. We remembered that as followers of Jesus, we'd been revived, regenerated, and delivered from the dark state in which so many of us still live.

With the guidance of the Holy Spirit, my zeal for ministry was reignited, burning afresh. Together, Brittany and I pulled ourselves out of our pit, having in common a renewed passion to serve God, a deep conviction to be led by the Holy Spirit, and a fiery commitment to walk in the light as He is in the light (1 John 1:7). When we finally became husband and wife, we were excited at the opportunity to be used by God, but we had no clue what that looked like. All I knew was that I didn't want to end up being good at a whole bunch of things. I felt like God was calling me to be great at just one thing. When I told Brittany, she said, "Me, too!"

So I said, "Okay, what does that look like?" We shrugged our shoulders because we both had no idea. But our priorities were definitely what they needed to be—God, the church, our family. We both wanted a life centered on God, service to the church, and love for family. At the start of our marriage, I was managing a small bar and grill not far from where we lived. As we were praying and seeking direction, God provided an opportunity for me to be done with the nightlife and pursue a career in an industry Brittany and I had grown to love: fitness. It also made sense to us because we had met in the gym.

A significant portion of our friendship was cultivated on a mutual desire to be healthy and fit since both of us had testimonies of being very out of shape more than enough times in our lives. After we made the decision to become personal trainers, our passion for fitness became obvious. We loved being part of people's journeys on the uphill climb to more energy, more confidence, and more strength. We were definitely inspired as we learned together, grew together, and consistently motivated each other.

One night during a personal training session with my friend and brother in Christ, James Cook, we struck up a conversation about the mission field. I had never been on an international missions trip, so I was intrigued by everything James had to say about it. He expressed a concern that over the years, something in missions work had been lost. Christians were experiencing long-term exhaustion and suffering from diminished interest. Some were devoted in duty but lacked joy and were now just going through the motions. Others sought to change the face of missions into something that could be fun, relaxing, and comfortable instead of what had typically been tough and strenuous.

I agree that missions work isn't a vacation; it's supposed to be uncomfortable. It's about getting in the trenches with people in the midst of their problems, unprotected by distance or illusion. Ministry should be down and dirty, not cushy and cozy. The scripture that came to my mind during our conversation that night was a direct quote from Jesus.

If anyone would come after me, let him deny himself and take up his cross daily and follow me.

—Luke 9:23

And there it was! In that moment, I knew that Christians, myself included, were fast becoming a people who don't mind following Jesus but had found a way to do it without denying ourselves and without taking up our crosses. In short, we're missing the mark in this daily charge. I asked myself, *What does it look like to serve God sacrificially, wholeheartedly, and unashamedly?*

I wanted to know where I was missing the mark and settling for a lukewarm faith in Christ. I needed to know for myself if I was on fire for God or if I was minimally giving my life to Jesus who has maximally given His all to me.

I thought that surely there are numerous stumbling blocks and spiritual barriers I encounter and struggle with every day. But what about the physical ones? I never thought about the connection between spiritual and physical fitness. I wondered if we should pay more attention to the physical health and wellness of the church. On Sundays, we hear exhortations from the pulpit about the struggle with lack of faith, lack of joy, and all things pertaining to spiritual warfare. But what about the battle of the body? What about the obesity, anorexia, diabetes, and high blood pressure that is crippling the body of Christ? How can we expect to give our all to God spiritually if we aren't getting equipped for all God has for us physically?

According to the US National Institutes of Health, two out of of three adults are considered overweight or obese.[1] That makes it

---

1. "Overweight & Obesity Statistics," *National Institute of Diabetes and Digestive and Kidney Diseases*, https://www.niddk.nih.gov/health-information/health-statistics/overweight-obesity.

easy to believe that there is somewhere around five Christians in every local church who are discouraged physically. They're not participating in enough missions or ministry because they're too out of shape or lack the confidence and strength to do so. The ones who are participating are getting burned out by the shortage of strong people, more specifically strong men. A lot of husbands are traveling for work, on the road eating fast food and ordering room service. The young men are back at home playing video games, and the wives, mothers, and daughters seem to be getting ministry done.

What if I told you that in addition to the five physically discouraged Christians in every church, there's an average of five more who are just plain lazy. When we multiply 10 Christians times 300,000 churches nationwide, we come up with about three million Christians. This number represents a huge epidemic and an issue of catastrophic proportions. Think of the worldwide effect if three million more Christians were vibrantly helping spread the gospel. Think about how much they would energize worship, invigorate generosity, and animate fellowship within our communities.

How many more Christians would travel to Haiti, Africa, China, and other countries if they were in better shape, had more energy, and had a stronger drive to serve the nations? What if we could help each other lose excess weight—10 to 30 pounds, or even 40 to 50— and get off our meds, inspiring each other into more ministry? And what if the dedication and discipline involved in diet and exercise could help improve our marriages, make us better parents, and bring forth revival? These are the questions Brittany and I started asking ourselves.

We both began to believe that fitness doesn't start with a doctor's orders or a mutual aid group, a broken arm or a broken relationship.

It doesn't start with a documentary on processed foods or a miracle pill from Dr. Oz. And it doesn't start with ourselves, either. It starts with God. The best place to begin a healthy lifestyle isn't in the gym but in the word of God—the Bible.

Here is the next question we asked ourselves: Is this biblical? Do we see Jesus making people stronger and healthier? The answer is yes. Meeting peoples' physical needs was a huge part of Jesus's ministry. Once we found the idea in scripture, Brittany and I launched the Faith-Infused Training Project—FIT Project for short. We believe that health and fitness should be pursued through the leadership of the Holy Spirit and carried out in a Christ-like manner.

We want to see the people of God, all Christians, be trained, equipped, and sent out into the world with the energy of God's spirit and the enthusiasm of Jesus. Our hope is to apply what we've learned, both in our study of fitness and our study of scripture, for the benefit of Christians everywhere. If we can motivate each other to attain stronger legs and arms through the strength of Christ, have healthier hearts filled with God's love and holiness, together we can stand firm as the body of Christ. If we can help Christians build stronger bone density upon the firm foundation of Jesus, improve cardiovascular systems to fight the good fight of faith, we can participate in the furtherance of the gospel with Christ-like power, bringing glory to God everywhere we go. What you will find in this book can do exactly that.

CHAPTER 1

Fitness Begins with Theology

As a family man, I have known and interacted with several parents who have joyously brought babies into this world. During their expecting stages, they would purchase clothes for newborns that have phrases like "I Love My Daddy" and "Mommy's Little Helper" on them. I wondered how they could know that these statements would be true of their kids. Perhaps it's just common for moms and dads to hope so. Or maybe they planned to pour reciprocal love into their children and teach them the responsibility of lending a hand around the house.

Throughout the infant and toddler stages, these parents also dialogued about which family genes seemed to be more dominant and whose faces their children resembled most, making statements like "She has her father's eyes but her mother's nose." No doubt, it is clearly evident that to conceive and give birth is to procreate in our image. And to raise a child, is to imprint on them our ideological standards for the purpose of passing on certain values. But where did that desire come from, and how did it start? Why do some believe it is necessary?

Where It All Began

Our makeup is the result of a unique and prolific design. Each of us is one-of-a-kind in body and soul. So, if you don't already, view yourself as exceptional. And collectively, we are the offspring of God our maker, traced all the way back to the first human beings who walked the earth, Adam and Eve. Every one of our family trees begins with this couple.

> *The man called his wife's name Eve, because she was the mother of all living.*
>
> —Gen. 3:20

We have all been created in the image of God. Those of us who are followers of Jesus, represent the adopted sons and daughters of the extended family of faith. As God's children, we are to love Him as father (creator) and produce life (results) for good. In essence, we are to bear His family name by exemplifying Him in every way possible—physically and spiritually, bodily and mentally; that is the nature of our existence.

But some of us seldom think about it that way. When we look in the mirror, it's hard to see past the resemblance of our fathers and mothers, our grandparents and great grandparents. It's easy to be a chip off the old block or an apple that doesn't fall far from the tree. Most of us are lovers of patterns and tend to safeguard our traditions, our routines, and our simplicity. We're proud of the places where we were born and raised, and we celebrate our nationalities and heritage frequently. Good times are a huge priority for us as our goal is to have a "normal" life.

On the other hand, some of us don't like what we see. Some of us are unhappy with our family name and the bodies we have to live in. We wish we could change who we are or perhaps where we came from, feeling underprivileged in the midst of those who are well-off. We're bitter at the fact that some guys inherit good genetics, dreamy eyes, and a perfect physique, while others get stuck with orangutan-type features. We get caught up in thinking how unfair it is that some girls are passed down a slender and balanced body, while others are bottom-heavy and stumpy.

As a Christian man, I definitely relate to all that. For the longest time, I thought I wouldn't amount to much because my ears were too big, and my hair wasn't cool enough. Pretty silly, huh? Such obstacles are an illusion and should have no bearing on our pursuit of happiness and well-being, which is directly connected to our health and fitness. At heart, I used to be a mile wide and an inch deep. I had never explored my reflection of the image of God or what it meant to live in light of His goodness. What I found is that living in harmony with His will and being able-bodied for His glory are the first steps in pursuing true health and ultimate transformation.

Fitness Begins with God

So if God is spirit, what does it mean to be physically created in His image? If He is invisible, why does the Bible ascribe somatic attributes to Him such as His strong arm, mighty hand, and all-seeing eyes? The shadow of His wings, the speaking of His mouth, the hearing of His ears—are those just elaborate attempts at anthropomorphism? Or is there a higher purpose and deeper meaning to our anatomy? And if so, does it matter what we do with our physical bodies? Does it matter what we eat or drink? Is it all the same to be brutishly fit or hoggishly fat? Should we even care?

The image of God is such a thought-engendering reflection that once considered, we discover its definition extends far beyond what we see and therefore compels a reverent honor toward our master builder. If it is He who gave us a body and a brain, then we should exert ourselves to take care of it. If it is He who gave us our lungs, our heart, and our liver, then we should protect them from harm. If our bodies have, in fact, been architected, we ought to protect their structure with strong muscles, healthy bones, and unblocked pathways toward exuberance.

Our unseen attitudes matter just as much as our measurable body fat. Our beating hearts are as important as our intangible minds. Our muscles and our midsections are to be cared for in a sacred manner, as are our words and our deeds. God made us in His image so we could mirror His strength, His endurance, and His quality of life. And if we humans are capable of being nurturers, how much more can all-powerful God provide everything to cultivate our relationship with Him? If we who are parents possess the ability to love and instruct our kids, how much more capable is an everlasting father like God.

Fitness Begins with Trusting God

Too often, I lived looking straight ahead, merely at the things around me and never bothering to look upward at the one watching over me. I continually struggled to find direction in life, sometimes lost without a cause avoiding the hard questions, and keeping myself distracted by comfort and entertainment. To preserve my sanity, I devoted myself to consumerism and capitalism by making as much money as I could to buy all the things I wanted. Me, myself, and I were united in our pursuit of self-gratification and fulfillment. I used to strive toward secularism and "peace," taking the stance that God was irrelevant in determining how we live.

As Christians, we know that nothing could be further from the truth. God should always be at the center of our lives with Christ at the center of our hearts. Arguably, it seems that many people blame religion for the interruption of the world's good times and consider it a damper on their good vibes. It does seem as if spiritual folks make things awkward with their hyperspirituality, abnormal clothes, vegetarian vows, picket signs, protests, and preachiness. Being governed by any religion is tough for a lot of people to accept.

Nonbelievers seem to feel like Christians are always judging them, and quite frankly, Christians haven't done a very good job of convincing them of the way, the truth, and the life. Sometimes, people can be overwhelmed by all the chaos and confusion in this world, making it easy for them to avoid God altogether. I'll be honest; I have sometimes fallen into a similar trap of doubt and unbelief. Mistrusting God, I developed my own principles and guidelines, set my own morals and values, and worked to get rich quick or die trying. I created bucket lists for myself, thinking life is lived between two hospitals—the one we're born in and the one that has our deathbed.

In the meantime, I looked out for myself and did what worked for me. My days as a kid were spent mostly in public classrooms getting educated and prepared for the "real world." I worked fast to find my identity and figure out what I wanted to do with this short life, making very little time for church because I'd much rather be watching football, making it a Sunday fun day. I was fascinated by discovery, but only in the natural sense, and I'd marvel at people's inventions rather than the creations of God. Social media and entertainment were my preferred sources of enlightenment. I lived in a world where relativism rules, self-image is sovereign, and postmodern culture prevails.

Fitness Calls for Godliness

If we want to be truly fit, we have to be godly. When we dismiss God's image and consign Him to oblivion, we become terribly unfamiliar with terms like *holiness* and remain estranged from godliness. We also soon forget that God is a king. His reign is over all, and as such, we must hold Him in the highest regard, treating Him as the highest being of most supreme royalty and authority. This idea resonates throughout all scripture.

> *Ascribe to the LORD the glory due his name; worship the LORD in the splendor of holiness.*
>
> —Ps. 29:2

God created us to always be under His care, to go to Him for everything we need. Spiritually and physically, God is our provider in all things.

> *May the LORD give strength to his people! May the LORD bless his people with peace!*
>
> —Ps. 29:11

God's motive is intentional out of love for us. Because He knows what's best for us, He offers no neutral stance to take, no independent party to join, and no overthrowing His government. God makes that very clear in His word.

> *Whoever is not with me is against me.*
>
> —Matt. 12:30

In order to begin to understand this, we must learn to think outside human logic and attempt to view life from His divine perspective. Instead of defining everything, seen and unseen, solely in accordance with a creature's perspective, we ought to analyze the mysteries that require biblical logic. For example, if God is our creator and father, then He is responsible for our lives. We are connected to Him in the same way that parents are connected to their children.

That connection consists of essentials, one of them being love. Just as parents love and care for their children, so God desires to love and care for us. As parents teach their children obedience and submission for their good, so God desires us to obey and healthily submit to Him for our good. Problems arise when we disobey, when we scorn, and when we go our own way.

Throughout this book, we will be examining Adam and Eve's story found in Genesis 3 of the Bible. One major reason is because Adam and Eve were the only two people alive before health issues existed. No one except Adam and Eve got to experience perfect bliss in its purest sense. That perfection had the power to provide a world without pain and frailty.

Imagine being alive and well as a 500-year-old man or woman with strong bones, impeccable skin, and the heart of a lion. Imagine running across the country without your feet hurting or even suffering a single shin splint. Picture being able to walk up flights of stairs without losing your breath or running up and down the bleachers of a stadium without your legs aching—ever.

What if you were able to play catch with your kids and never have shoulder issues, or lift weights all day and never experience soreness or the fear of muscle pulls? There was a time when we didn't have to worry about bad knees, back problems, arthritis, or multiple sclerosis. The world God created was full of never-ending joy, free from debilitation and enfeeblement. Adam and Eve were entrusted to be good stewards of all creation with 100 percent godliness. Needless to say, they were unsuccessful.

Prior to Adam and Eve being led astray by Satan and physically defying God, there wasn't even a hint of sickness on earth, no obesity, cancer, diabetes, or heart disease. As soon as Adam and Eve ate from the tree of the knowledge of good and evil, improper diet and poor decision-making entered the world. The moment they lost sight of God's particular instruction, the hereditary path to selfish craving and gluttony opened up to all humankind.

Fitness Requires Righteousness

When Adam and Eve went their own way and infringed upon the paradisiacal order, their union with God was severed. The realm of flesh declared war on the spiritual realm, and the dark existence of evil in the angelic realm was revealed. The perfect couple allowed themselves to be corrupted.

> *Now the serpent was more crafty than any other beast of the field that the LORD God had made. He said to the woman, "Did God actually say, 'You shall not eat of any tree in the garden'?"*

—Gen. 3:1

The serpent, Satan, caused Adam and Eve to question God's authority over their bodies, their overall health, and the wellness of their minds and souls. He convinced them of the lie that God was restricting their freedom when, in fact, God was protecting their dominion over the natural world.

> *But the serpent said to the woman, "You will not surely die. For God knows that when you eat of it your eyes will be opened, and you will be like God, knowing good and evil."*

—Gen. 3:4–5

This was the earliest instance of twisting God's words, and Eve fell victim to it. Instead of holding fast to her original interpretation of God's law as wholesome and secure, she took it upon herself to eat according to her own dietary guidelines and then fed her husband, Adam, who ate willingly against the standard of God's righteousness. For the first time on earth, there was an unhealthy situation. This circumstance produced emotional and physical repercussions to all and in all.

Adam and Eve were so ashamed of their disobedience that they hid themselves from God like two little kids who just made a mess and were about to be in trouble. This childish behavior continued as they pointed fingers and sought to shift blame. But God held them completely accountable by disciplining them and training them, just like a loving father would.

> *To the woman he said, "I will surely multiply your pain in childbearing; in pain you shall bring forth children. Your desire shall be contrary to your husband, and he shall rule over you." And to Adam he said, "Because you have listened to the voice of your wife and have eaten of the tree of which I commanded you, 'You shall not eat of it,' cursed is the ground because of you; in pain you shall eat of it all the days of your life; thorns and thistles it shall bring forth for you; and you shall eat the plants of the field. By the sweat of your face you shall eat bread, till you return to the ground, for out of it you were taken; for you are dust, and to dust you shall return."*
>
> —Gen. 3:16–19

God, promising to remedy iniquity, also announced the coming of justice through His son, who would carry the sword of recompense for those against Him but the message of mercy for those who are with Him.

> *The LORD God said to the serpent, "Because you have done this, cursed are you above all livestock and above all the beasts of the field; . . . I will*

put enmity between you and the woman, and between your offspring and her offspring; he shall bruise your head and you shall bruise his heel."

—Gen. 3:14–15

From that point on, every child born came into the world through pain, stained by this corruption, and all of life would be affected by it. To this day, we are feeling the affliction caused by disobedience as life gets challenging, overwhelming, and difficult. Our bodies suffer from pain and stress, demoralization and depression. It's an unavoidable pain whether we're fit or unfit, existing in both the lazy and the active and among those who overeat and those who diet. That is why we need Jesus, the sinless savior, because everyone, like Adam and Eve, will inevitably succumb to self-will.

For our sake he made him to be sin who knew no sin, so that in him we might become the righteousness of God.

—2 Cor. 5:21

It makes you wonder why complete obedience was required in the first place. Why even afford the opportunity to disobey? Doesn't it seem like God overreacted a bit? Those are both serious questions to ask. But it's difficult to understand the will of an omniscient God when we as finite humans define life how we see fit rather than how He sees it. Once we get to know God and become more familiar with who He is, we will better understand His infinitely profound mind and His perfect ways.

What we can conclude from God's reaction is that He desires for us to live life as He instructs us in all things. Everything in creation was perfect until Adam and Eve disregarded God's commandment for something that was unsanctioned and untrue. Through a short-lived moment of satisfied hunger and selfish ambition, Adam and Eve's anxiety, insecurity, and guilt cast a dark shadow on the human race, resulting in three emergent factors in today's eating disorders.

Health and fitness should be pursued by getting our bodies right with God with godly ambition, by contentment in Christ, and through the confidence of the Holy Spirit. When our actions reflect that we trust what God says, it is called faith.

> *By faith we understand that the universe was created by the word of God, so that what is seen was not made out of things that are visible.*
> —Heb. 11:3

Not everything real is visible. Not all power is to be found here on earth and restricted to humans. There is a power we have not yet seen face-to-face, a king enthroned in heaven through whom all things came to be by the word of His mouth (Ps. 33:9). His very breath gave all of us life (Genesis 2:7). This power is what gives God the authority to determine what is good and what is bad, and by faith, we submit to how He lovingly governs and wisely rules our lives.

Sin Produces Unhealthiness

In the mind of God, who established good, all wrongdoing is equally offensive because it all stems from contention with Him. Whether it's a forbidden tree or forbidden thoughts and actions, each is punished the same—by death. I used to think that all wrongdoing existed on a top-to-bottom list, from minor and tolerable to heinous and unacceptable. For example, before I got married, I worked long, hard weeks and then went out and treated myself over the weekend. I splurged, got stinking drunk, and overate a ton. As long as I was responsible, I thought it was okay.

What I needed to realize was that in the eyes of a holy God, drunkenness to any degree, carelessness, addiction, and gluttony are all equally punishable. The main reason is that all these behaviors go against every attribute of God's character and violate every aspect of His divine nature. God has never done anything wrong. He's perfectly sinless, and He has never transgressed. Nothing in God's ways portrays Him as gluttonous, slothful, or lacking in self-control. Wrongdoing is not in Him at all. So when the world, which He created, participates in things that aren't good, it shatters every aspect of His image.

History displays our increasing tolerance for unhealthiness in a way that really doesn't leave any of us exempt. The result: We do as we please and chase what we crave, no matter what the cost or consequence. Right now, illegal drugs are far more available and popular among a now wider spectrum of adolescents to adults. Each year, drunkenness and alcohol abuse are steadily on the rise among youth and the elderly. Men are spending less time on the grill and women less time at the stove because there's more fast food available to eat and more restaurants to go to. At the push of a button, we can even have our favorite fattening junk delivered right to our doorstep.

Today, our world suffers from disease and decay, from minor strokes to massive heart attacks, kidney failure, malnutrition, emotional eating, and stress drinking. All of those exist as a result of the transgression of divine law. We can never truly accomplish a life that reflects God's perfect image, which is why we need a healthy relationship with the perfect son of God, Jesus. But the straight and narrow path has been ignored without exception by many who have forsaken biblical principles. To a certain degree, we have all forgotten God or denied our originator at one time or another. Some have even replaced Him with Big Bang theories and Mother Nature, resorting to atheistic and agnostic views, just to name a few.

God Makes Health and Fitness Possible

If God intended to rule with righteousness over a perfect and healthy people, why did He give us free will? He did that so we can know our decisions have real meaning and therefore carry with them real consequences. Free will informs us that we can't blame God or anyone else for the health and condition of our lives. The responsibility is ours, and we are the ones who should be held accountable. But God isn't just the judge and ruler over all things. He is, in fact, the creator of all things and the giver of all things, righteous in all ways. His purpose is always good, no matter how bad life gets. His actions are forever in the best interest of Himself, His son, His spirit, His kingdom, and His people.

Now that we have discovered together that God gives, we can also agree that we receive. Every day we receive, because every day God gives. Each time you breathe in and out, you receive God-given air for your lungs. Every day you spend on this planet, you receive your God-given gift of life. Every time you look or watch with your eyes—everything you see—you see it with the sight that God gave you. Whenever you eat vegetables, fruit, or meat, you receive God's gift of food to humankind. You see, my friends, God is everywhere. And our free will is the means by which we experience and embrace His blessings.

Think back on your children (or on your parents, if you have no kids). We seek to give our children comfort, nourishment, food, and shelter. Thus, they are the recipients of our provision. They bear the image of our natural love and care. Likewise, we all bear the image of God's heavenly endowment and His boundless benevolence. As we seek to contribute humanely to our families, to society, and to the environment, so God contributes by upholding the universe, sustaining the earth, and conserving our livelihood.

God Takes Action Spiritually and Physically

The Bible is the testimony of God's conservation, primarily in the spiritual sense, but most certainly in the physical sense, because God goes to great lengths to preserve the state of our physical lives. He makes commitments to His people using unbreakable promises called covenants. One of those covenants was with a man named Abraham, a great patriarch of faith whom God called to be the father of many nations.

> *I am God Almighty; walk before me, and be blameless, that I may make my covenant between me and you, and may multiply you greatly. . . . Behold, my covenant is with you . . . Abraham, for I have made you the father of a multitude of nations. I will make you exceedingly fruitful . . . and your offspring after you throughout their generations for an everlasting covenant . . . and I will be their God.*
>
> —Gen. 17:1–2,4–8

Abraham was called by God, and throughout his story, we see a hedge of physical protection over him, like in battle.

> *When Abram heard that his kinsman had been taken captive, he led forth his trained men. . . . And he divided his forces against them by night, he and his servants, and defeated them. . . . Then he brought back . . . his kinsman Lot with his possessions, and the women and the people.*
>
> —Gen. 14:14–16

Abraham had guts, he had strength, and he had strategy. But most of all, and most necessary, he had God who was his strength.

Blessed be Abram by God Most High, Possessor of heaven and earth; and blessed be God Most High, who has delivered your enemies into your hand!

—Gen. 14:19–20

God's unbreakable promises continued throughout Moses's days. It was God's strong arm and outstretched hand that overthrew Pharaoh and rescued God's people out of Egypt.

To Him who divided the Red Sea in two . . . and made Israel pass through the midst of it . . . but overthrew Pharaoh and his host in the Red Sea, for His steadfast love endures forever.

—Ps. 136:13–15

As Moses led God's people into the wilderness, it was through God's providential power that He turned bitter water into sweet.

When they came to Marah, they could not drink the water of Marah because it was bitter. . . . And the people grumbled against Moses. . . . And he cried to the LORD, and the LORD showed him a log, and he threw it into the water, and the water became sweet.

—Exod. 15:23–25

God also rained down bread from heaven and brought quail into their camp to eat.

*And the LORD said to Moses . . . "At twilight **you shall eat meat**, and in the morning **you shall be filled with bread**. Then **you shall know that I am the LORD your God**."*

—Exod. 16:11–12

In Moses's battles, it was the staff of God that protected them from defeat, giving them strength to overcome weakness and guaranteeing victory.

> So Moses said to Joshua, "**Choose for us men, and go out and fight** with Amalek. Tomorrow I will stand on the top of the hill **with the staff of God in my hand**." So Joshua did as Moses told him, and fought with Amalek.... Whenever Moses held up his hand, **Israel prevailed**.... So his hands were steady until the going down of the sun. And **Joshua overwhelmed Amalek and his people with the sword**.
>
> —Exod. 17:9–13

Throughout the Old Testament, we see God providing physical protection and deliverance for His people. Although His perfect image has been shattered by sin on earth, God desires to safeguard the broken pieces, which are us, until the time when His image will be perfectly restored. That is what the New Testament is all about—the mirror image of God in the face of Christ and the life of Christ manifested in the bodies of His people.

> For God, who said, "Let light shine out of darkness," has shone in our hearts to give the light of the knowledge of the glory of God in the face of Jesus Christ. But we have this treasure in jars of clay, to show that the surpassing power belongs to God and not to us.
>
> —2 Cor. 4:6–7

In everything physical, God is not simply behind the scenes, nor is He a passive spectator. No, He shepherds us, hears our requests, speaks to us, and creates the spiritual and physical path of greatness for our good. So yes, it does matter what we do with our bodies. Our physical capabilities and limitations are important to God because we are made in His image both internally and externally. His image is in our chests, our hands, our feet, our backs, and our faces. Our bodies were designed to clearly show a family delineation to God in the form of the light of Jesus Christ, who is our righteousness.

> *Do not present your members to sin as instruments for unrighteousness,*
> *but present yourselves to God as those who have been brought from death*
> *to life, and your members to God as instruments for righteousness.*
> —Romans 6:13

We Need God-Centered Fitness

What we do with our bodies begins with the image of God. What we eat and what we drink should be decided by our connection to Him. God is Spirit, yes, but He is also concerned with the physical. We are physical beings, but the choices we make should be based on spiritual things that matter to God because fitness takes on many other forms than just how it pertains to our bodies. Abraham was fit to be known as the father of faith because he worshipped God and trusted Him with his whole life. Moses was fit to lead Israel out of captivity because he believed God and submitted to God's mission. Jesus is fit to be at the right hand of God, having lived a perfect life, fulfilling God's purpose without a single flaw in His mind, body, or soul.

I used to think of fitness as just physical. I'd go straight to anatomy and the science of it all. I'd think of bulging biceps, rock-hard abs, and massive legs. I'd picture well-balanced meals high in protein, low in fat, with moderate carbs and a glass of skim milk. I'd assume cardio, weight lifting, plyometrics, and stretching exercises were involved. Those might be accurate assessments, but it's only half the battle in the body.

The rest of the fight for fitness is spiritual, deep down in our souls, as it applies to all areas of our lives. The condition and health of our souls determine how far we will climb to succeed at work, at home, and at play. To instill the discipline of fitness in the body, we must first access the mind God gave us through His Holy Spirit. Our outlook should always be through the lens of biblical theology, because at the peak of the mountain of muscle gain is God our creator, and the light at the end of the weight-loss tunnel is Jesus our savior. In Him is our truest gain, our truest victory.

CHAPTER 2
Be Strong in Christ

The only person to ever flawlessly manifest the image of God on earth is Jesus. In every inch of his body, inside and out, God's presence perfectly dwelt. His DNA was the molecular blueprint of the alpha and the omega. His brain was immersed in the thoughts of our Lord, His face filled with the glory of God. Almighty strength bound every intricate fiber of His muscle. His heart pumped the blood of eternal life; His eyes and ears were all-seeing and all-hearing. Scripture heralds Him as the source of all humanity, the mightiest of heroes, and foremost in all strength.

> *He is the image of the invisible God, the firstborn of all creation. For by him all things were created, in heaven and on earth, visible and invisible, whether thrones or dominions or rulers or authorities—all things were created through him and for him . . . and in him all things hold together. And he is the head of the body, the church. He is the beginning . . . that in everything he might be preeminent. For in him all the fullness of God was pleased to dwell, and through him to reconcile to himself all things, whether on earth or in heaven, making peace by the blood of his cross.*
> —Col. 1:15–20

Jesus had amazing supernatural strength throughout His entire body. By the power of His mouth He cast out demons, raised people from the dead, and made paralytics walk. With a single touch, He brought physical healing to deformities, blindness, and leprosy. With open arms, He embraced our due punishment on His back and carried the heavy burden of our sin on His shoulders. With His hands and feet, He paid our debt to God, holding nothing back, sparing no expense, to bring us our greatest gift and fulfill our greatest need.

> *For all have sinned and fall short of the glory of God, and are justified*
> *by his grace as a gift, through the redemption that is in Christ Jesus.*
>
> —Rom. 3:23–24

Jesus Is Our Strength

What is our greatest need? Is it water? Is it air? Is it food, sex, or money? Our greatest need is what has been provided for us by the one who is greatest. And the one who is greatest is God, who has freely given us His son. Without Jesus, there is no water, no air, no food, no source of pleasure, and no serenity or security. Our greatest need is God as lord and savior, through whom our physical bodies are restored in this life and in the next.

This truth serves as a foundation for spiritual contentment, but also for physical contentment. Whether you're shaped like a toothpick or fluffy like a marshmallow, only Jesus can provide you with the purest form of peace and happiness. Whether you're trying hard to bulk up or lose weight, be a model or an athlete, only Jesus can provide you with the purest form of steadfastness and perseverance.

Probably one of the most quoted New Testament verses is about achieving goals through Jesus and responding to Him as our chief essential for fitness:

> *I can do all things through him who strengthens me.*
>
> —Phil. 4:13

It's awesome when we have the word of God on our minds during training and competition. Reciting scripture and meditating on it while we walk, run, lift, bike, or swim is an invaluable part of growing in faith and in strength. But being fit doesn't magically happen for God's people. It requires energy, effort, focus, and hard work. Can the strength of Christ empower us physically? Absolutely! But primarily, the strength of Christ teaches us to beautifully display gladness in all circumstances.

So whether our stats are incredible or our fitness records embarrassing, our strength is in Him, not in ourselves. Whether we can do 50 pull-ups or zero pull-ups, our hearts and minds should be at ease, knowing that physical toughness comes in time from disciplined training. Being filled with joy through the process brings Christ-like inspiration to all and a sweet-smelling aroma of glory to God. That sets us up to be like Jesus in humility, suffering, devotion, and stewardship. Then, in due time, we can flourish, grow, and become die-hard in Christ.

God Is Jesus's Strength

How strong was Jesus? Was He able to do all things through God who strengthened Him? While we can only guess what the workout habits of Jesus were, we can believe that by the time he was 12 years old, He had become fit.

> *And the child grew and became strong, filled with wisdom. And the favor of God was upon Him.*
>
> —Luke 2:40

We read in the Bible that everything Jesus possessed, in his mind and in his body, increased by having favor with God. By the time He was a grown man, He was well-versed in scripture and well-liked by those around Him. Physically, Jesus had to have been in the best shape of His life, doing strenuous construction work throughout the years and walking everywhere. He maintained a well-balanced whole foods diet, eating in moderation, according to Jewish custom. He also had full self-control. He fasted for 40 days prior to beginning His ministry, a journey that consisted of hiking up mountains, back and forth through hills and difficult slopes.

We also know that a greater hedge of physical protection was upon Jesus in the perfect anatomy and strength of the Holy Spirit.

> *The Holy Spirit descended on him in bodily form, like a dove; and a voice came from heaven, "You are my beloved Son; with you I am well pleased."*
>
> —Luke 3:22

Just as in the case of Moses and Abraham, God's spiritual intervention was required in the life and ministry of Jesus. It provided enough physical protection for Him to carry out His mission with unparalleled success.

> *Because you have made the LORD your dwelling place—the Most High, who is my refuge—no evil shall be allowed to befall you, no plague come near your tent. For he will command his angels concerning you to guard you in all your ways. On their hands they will bear you up, lest you strike your foot against a stone.*
>
> —Ps. 91:9–12

In the early part of Jesus's ministry, He was tempted by the devil under physically demanding circumstances. Jesus hadn't eaten in more than a month. He was hungry, tired, and vulnerable. The devil literally quoted Psalm 91 to get Jesus to jump off a building and commit suicide. At the highest point of the temple in Jerusalem he said to Jesus,

If you are the Son of God, throw yourself down from here.
—Luke 4:9

Jesus, exhausted from physical and emotional strain, answered back with the word of God that served as His "food" during that time.

You shall not put the Lord your God to the test.
—Luke 4:12

Strength Serves Great Purpose

Jesus dealt with His physical and emotional challenges by quoting scripture and taking refuge and comfort in God, who is forever our shield. This set the example of how all of us should respond to adversity. The devil, knowing Jesus had been sent by God to conquer evil, treated Jesus as any other human in the flesh, just as he did with Eve in the Garden of Eden. The devil's plan is always to kill us spiritually and destroy us physically.

Jesus knew the devil was trying to trick Him. He also knew the solution to his momentary affliction was not to put an end to His own suffering by jumping off a ledge. Giving into temptation was never an option for Jesus. He proved that to the devil's face, demonstrating the strength and power of God's word by carrying on in His plan to restore us spiritually and revive us physically.

So often, we face these same challenges and temptations. It seems as though our challenges never end. Work gets tough, relationships get tough, and the pressure is on financially, emotionally, and physically. We have the perfect model in Jesus to knock out the stress in our minds, body-slam the addiction in our hearts, and shot-put the devil's influence out of our souls. But too many of us would rather eat, drink, and smoke our cares away. We'd rather numb our pain with sedatives, alcohol, and comfort foods. When we do that at an unhealthy rate, in overconsumption, we become fit for the devil's game and totally unfit for the prize in Jesus.

As a believer, I am certain I'm going to heaven when I die, but that doesn't mean I can draw relief from things that can kill me. Addictions to alcohol, fast food, painkillers, and black-market steroids once sent my health into a quick downward spiral. Alcoholism was killing me, high cholesterol was killing me, obesity was killing me, and pretty much all things unhealthy were killing me. The devil was slowly asking me to throw myself off a cliff. Because of the example of Jesus, my answer was most definitely no. So if we are ever tempted to put things in our bodies that cripple or slowly kill us, the Christ-like thing to do is to resist at all costs.

There is more to being human than the wild adrenaline rush of reckless behavior or the thrill of heart-pounding entertainment while living on the edge. We should also pay attention to more than just the haphazardly mundane, the eyebrow-raising coincidences, unexpected chance, and lucky days. God has a plan for our lives that is fitting for our ultimate destination—His kingdom of true paradise, the place where we will live forever without pain, fear, or doubt. There will be no frailty—only strength, never-ending happiness, and excellence.

What I am saying is that in all things, we must carry on according to the master's precepts, as Jesus did, in the likeness of His father, our creator. We must learn to trust fully in God, never forgetting that He does all things with perfect patience, in perfect timing, with perfect order, and through perfect strength.

> *We rejoice in our sufferings, knowing that suffering produces endurance, and endurance produces character, and character produces hope, and hope does not put us to shame, because God's love has been poured into our hearts through the Holy Spirit who has been given to us. For while we were still weak, at the right time Christ died for the ungodly.*
>
> —Rom. 5:3–6

Just as important as the fact that Jesus had physical strength is the fact that God's timing for His existence on earth was impeccable. Jesus appeared on the scene in the fullness of time. Every detail about the generation into which He was born was necessary for His life and death. From the virgin Mary to the cross on calvary, God called the shots perfectly in Jesus. He couldn't have been born any earlier or later. There were specific reasons why he was born in the lowly town of Bethlehem and why He started His ministry in His 30s, not when He was 40 or 50. He had to be rejected by His own people, received by Gentile sinners, and crucified by a Roman Empire.

Sovereign Strategy and Strength

What are the special details of your life? You were born to a specific mother and father in a specific place, just as Jesus was. God designed everything about you, from your genes to your family upbringing. He placed you here for a purpose. He positions all of us with the ability to think and act. He gives us ears so that when He speaks, we hear His direction and can fulfill our calling to pursue our destiny. The road isn't always smooth. But as long as we make ourselves fit to walk in His ways, God strategically prepares in advance His victorious outcome in every situation, good or bad.

> *Delight yourself in the LORD, and he will give you the desires of your heart. Commit your way to the LORD; trust in him, and he will act.*
>
> —Ps. 37:4–5

Throughout biblical history, God has been taking action. It was God who brought the first physical family unit together.

> *And the rib that the LORD God had taken from the man he made into a woman and brought her to the man.... Therefore a man shall leave his father and his mother and hold fast to his wife, and they shall become one flesh.*
>
> —Gen. 2:22, 24

From that point on, God has been the remedy in the fight for His people's fitness, the solution to unhealthiness and physical affliction. It was God who initiated the building of Noah's ark to preserve Noah and his family from the flood (1 Pet. 3:20). It was God who freed His own people from slavery and from the tyranny of the Egyptians (Exod. 14:30–31). When Job suffered at the hands of Satan (Job 1:8–12), it was God who restored him with lifelong comfort, joy, and fortune (Job 42:10–17). It was God who ordained the birth of Jesus (Luke 1:30–31), authorized His life and ministry (John 5:19), endured His sacrificial death, and then seated Him at His right hand as king.

> *And being found in human form, he humbled himself by becoming obedient to the point of death, even death on a cross. Therefore God has highly exalted him and bestowed on him the name that is above every name, so that at the name of Jesus every knee should bow, in heaven and on earth and under the earth, and every tongue confess that Jesus Christ is Lord, to the glory of God the Father.*
>
> —Phil. 2:8–11

This pansophical, loving God likewise brought you into this world, fashioned for you a body to experience His goodness through thick and thin to reveal Himself as father and creator of all. He provided a way for you to be saved by His son, the redeemer of all.

> *For we are his workmanship, created in Christ Jesus for good works, which God prepared beforehand, that we should walk in them.*
> —Eph. 2:10

God's Order Demonstrates Strength

Each one of us has a purpose to fulfill, and it requires that we be strong in the Lord. Every female has a responsibility to "woman up," and the guys need to "man up." The same was true of Jesus, as His objective in life required physical endurance in all things. It demanded all His time, effort, and perfection in all things. It involved pain and heartache, zealous anger, and longsuffering, but in the end, there was joy and peace. It warranted stamina, bravery, resolve, blood, sweat, and tears, but in the end, there was glory and victory. Jesus's body and blood were both paramount in His ultimate sacrifice to carry out God's will. His life and death, both preeminent in society, were beautifully orchestrated to bring God's mission to completion. Jesus's life also necessitated a meticulous game plan, including key individuals such as John the Baptist, an ordained messenger of the coming Messiah (Luke 1:13–17). There was also Peter, appointed by Jesus on which He would build the church.

> *And I tell you, you are Peter, and on this rock I will build my church, and the gates of hell shall not prevail against it.*
> —Matt. 16:18

Later on, Paul was selected to evangelize the unreached world.

But the Lord said to him, "Go, for he is a chosen instrument of mine to carry my name before the Gentiles and kings and the children of Israel."
—Acts 9:15

These men were developed over time spiritually and physically by the strength of God and in the strength of Christ. God unfailingly chose for all of this to go down the way it did, in the time it did, and with the very men and women who were a part of His definitive mission. It all happened for a reason.

When we look more deeply into the unique facets of our own lives, we'll find that everything happens for a reason. The same was true beforehand, the same is true now, which means we were placed on earth in this specific time. If God had specific reasons and purposes to do that with everyone else, you can bet the same applies to us. Today, we can be sure God follows through on His work with staying power and at the perfect moment of strength and strategy.

It is believed that Jesus was about 30 years old, in His prime, when He began His ministry (Luke 3:23). As a child, though, at about the age of 12, He already possessed enough knowledge and wisdom to profess that He was the son of God (Luke 2:49). But He couldn't have started His ministry then. He hadn't even become a teacher or a spiritual leader yet and wouldn't have been accepted in the temple. And no one would have followed a kid or crucified a young boy on a cross for claiming to be the son of God.

On the other hand, if Jesus had waited until He was older, maybe 60, He would have been disregarded as a weak old man. His heart would have barely, if at all, been able to physically handle the rigorous terrain of Israel or escaping the men who were trying to kill him

(Luke 4:29–30 and John 10:39). Add to that the emotional shock and stress that caused Him hematidrosis (Luke 22:44), the beatings, the scourging, and the agonizing journey leading up to His crucifixion.

The timeline God chose showed me the many things I think I need today but actually don't. Jesus didn't need the spoils of a first-world country, but sometimes I seem to be helpless without them. I'm reliant on the comforts of air conditioning, hot water, and electricity. Jesus had none of those things and lived a perfect life. I like to hide behind emails, passive aggressive text messages, and social media. Jesus did everything face-to-face, and He was the greatest man to ever walk the earth.

Sometimes, I "need" processed foods or drinks to sustain me, but Jesus relied fully on the word of God for the foundation of His health. Spiritual nourishment enabled Him to complete all His tasks. I tend to dream of expensive sports cars, million-dollar mansions, a hefty retirement portfolio, fashion, and celebrity status. Jesus had everything He needed for life on earth, devoid of all those temporal things.

In certain past situations, I felt like I had to avoid offending people by minimizing conversations about God and faith, but Jesus didn't do that. He didn't launch what He stood for by blending in with political correctness or social acceptance. He was rejected by many who not only ignored His message but actively hated it because it deeply contradicted their lifestyles. Yet, His face was filled with determination, strong as a rock and covered in fearlessness.

But the Lord God helps me; therefore I have not been disgraced; therefore I have set my face like a flint, and I know that I shall not be put to shame. He who vindicates me is near. Who will contend with me? Let us stand up together. Who is my adversary? Let him come near to me.

—Isa. 50:7–8

It was prophesied that Jesus would be bold and courageous, putting Himself in harm's way and living radically for the sake of the truth, no matter what it cost Him. Jesus didn't need a normal life to validate His credibility. He wasn't dependent on a high social status, the support of elitists, a prestigious career, or a trophy wife. Nor did He need properties or capital to accomplish His ambition. His assets were love and humility. His hedge fund was comprised of ordinary fishermen, mostly nonprofessionals, and lower-class people, not hotshots. He invested in mercy and grace, and His return was power and glory.

Jesus's Fitness Demonstrates Power

Destined to be a ransom for many, a mediator between God and man, Jesus's body had to be fit, prepared to make it to the finish line—death on the cross.

> *Let us run with endurance the race that is set before us, looking to Jesus, the founder and perfecter of our faith, who for the joy that was set before him endured the cross, despising the shame, and is seated at the right hand of the throne of God.*
>
> —Heb. 12:1–2

His skin and bones were robust. Surely, God would not send His son unequipped to physically receive His wrath.

> *Trust in the LORD with all your heart, and do not lean on your own understanding. In all your ways acknowledge him, and he will make straight your paths. Be not wise in your own eyes; fear the LORD, and turn away from evil. It will be healing to your flesh and refreshment to your bones.*
>
> —Prov. 3:5–8

Think of it this way. What father whose son desires to be a champion wouldn't first teach him to win, provide him with coaching, and watch him practice long and hard before letting him take the field of play? What platoon leader whose trained soldiers are eager to win wars for their country wouldn't conduct a weapons check or inspect their gear for full functionality before letting them take the field of battle? How could God not dispense the necessary strength required to flawlessly execute His plan of salvation before letting His only begotten son sacrifice Himself for an entire people?

And there appeared to him an angel from heaven, strengthening him.
—Luke 22:43

This is all relevant to fitness. It matters how strong we are inside and out, how we overcome weakness, and how we seek His counsel to do so. Only when we see the creator's design in the very fabric of our bodies can we better make sound decisions pertaining to our mind, soul, and body. To be truly fit means to be like Jesus, who was steadfast in mind and in heart, perfectly strong from head to toe, in body and soul. He has been exalted as the highest, the greatest of all time, which is one reason He is still talked about thousands of years after His death. It's why thousands of years later, we still talk about His life. We celebrate His birth at Christmas and His resurrection at Easter every year. We regularly celebrate communion globally to commemorate His body and blood. That is the effect of a man who utterly commits his mind, body, and soul to the work of God. Just as God displays strength at all times for His glory, Jesus displayed strength at all times for God's glory, and so we must always emulate this example.

This commitment is something to consider beyond spring break and summertime. We should want to be in shape whether there's a wedding coming up or not, a beauty pageant to win or not. We ought to be fit for more reasons than physique contests, powerlifting tournaments, and running marathons.

Dress for Action

How are you preparing your body in the strength of Christ for the work of God? Throughout the history of God's people, it seems that the call to drop everything and follow Him could come at any time and last longer than expected. It took Noah decades to build the ark that preserved his family so the human race could live on after God flooded the earth. Joseph, whose story is found in the book of Genesis, was abandoned by his brothers, sold into slavery, and then spent years in prison for a crime he did not commit. After Joseph endured a rough physical journey, God made him a powerful ruler over the land of Egypt. Solomon, the son of King David, spent years of his life building a temple for God along with thousands of heavy lifters and craftsmen.

When the Jews of the prophet Nehemiah's day faced great trouble and shame, Nehemiah dedicated months laboring and rebuilding Jerusalem's wall. His efforts helped restore a whole city for many who were in physical and emotional distress. Paul the apostle, who did a lot of traveling, was shipwrecked a few times, falsely imprisoned, and persecuted by many. He took the beatings, endured the floggings, and was almost stoned to death. These men, like Jesus, trained for something far greater than themselves. Their heartfelt faith, which produced strength in them, was inspired by God.

Our created bodies belong to the one who created us. And if we are saved, our bodies belong to the one who has saved us—Jesus. When we embrace salvation, we inherit the desire to live actively for God, to be led spiritually by His son, and to meet the needs of others through the gospel. Only when we view ourselves through

God's eyes can we further understand what it means to be strong in Christ. We are part of a band of brothers and sisters, a family united to stand together, an army ready to defend righteousness and truth for Jesus's sake.

> *You then, my child, be strengthened by the grace that is in Christ Jesus, and what you have heard from me . . . entrust to faithful men, who will be able to teach others also. Share in suffering as a good soldier of Christ Jesus.*
> —2 Tim. 2:1–3

What do you see when you look at your body? Do you think of it as yours or as His? Do you see a randomly evolved specimen, or do you see a wonderfully made masterpiece? What do you see when Jesus Christ is displayed nailed to a cross? Do you see strength or weakness, justice or injustice, a wasted life or a sacrifice for humankind?

> *For there is one God, and there is one mediator between God and men, the man Christ Jesus, who gave himself as a ransom for all, which is the testimony given at the proper time.*
> —1 Tim. 2:5–6

Before I became aware that someone (Jesus) had died because of me, it was common for me to take a passive approach toward our compassionate redeemer. I halfheartedly took part in Him, who wholeheartedly gave all to us. Jesus is well-known by many as the man of sorrows who was wounded, beaten, and put to death, but not defeated. Yet it was so easy for me to overlook His amazing strength in spite of how He cast aside our weakness.

Our bodies were made for the glory and work of God. Our minds and souls were saved for the glory and work of Christ. There is no one on earth to be cherished more than Jesus and nothing to be vastly treasured above His truth. It is impossible to obsess too much about it. God's glory knows no bounds. His love transcends space and time forever and ever, reflecting infinite value. Jesus knew these truths which is how He was able to devote His all to God's big picture, to fulfill the grand scheme, and to be exceedingly happy to do so.

To be strong in Christ is to know exactly what to devote your body to and why, and to be disciplined enough to know how to bodily reflect that devotion. Being a Christian means pouring out our energy and enthusiasm for Christ's purposes, to gladly sweat, bleed, and even lay down our lives if He should require us to do so. God doesn't think in terms of this short life we only live once, and neither should we. We must think in terms of eternity, keeping our minds and bodies healthy, waiting in joyful hope for the certain return of our savior, Jesus Christ our strength.

CHAPTER 3

The Holy Spirit Empowers Us

In a world that cycles through times and seasons, from generations to eras, according to calendars and schedules, it's easy to think strictly in terms of beginnings and endings. Day begins at dawn and ends at sunset. School starts with kindergarten and finishes up at 12th grade graduation. College campus life begins with wormy freshmen and ends with stupendous college grads. Career paths start with ambitious rookies who work 40 hours per week for 40 years and then retire in style.

Our youth ends in old age, and inevitably, life expires at death. But for the Christian who has to think in terms of life after death, an uneasy struggle transpires. For us, God decides the beginnings and the endings, and as such, we don't really have the option of just going through the motions. We have the privilege of being responsible for discovering what is righteous and good, fruitful and meaningful, but by His definitions of those words, not ours. It then becomes necessary to consider how we should live in the sight of God as it pertains to all aspects of life, including health and fitness.

My life was a lot different when I made my own decisions based on how I felt or according to my circumstances. I see this throughout all my past. As a lazy student who never felt like studying or getting a tutor, I made it a habit to cheat my way to a high school diploma. As an impatient weightlifter who wanted quicker muscle gains, I felt like illegal steroids were the obvious route. When I was in sales, I couldn't make money fast enough, so I resorted to lies, deception, and fraud. These reasons and many more serve as long-lived examples of how we misuse and abuse our minds, bodies, and souls.

God Gives His Spirit for Our Bodies

As a follower of Christ, I don't really have the accommodation of doing whatever I feel is right all the time, although I thought I did. I would explode in anger, use foul language, grumble, and complain, even though the Bible spoke against those things. Even though everything I wanted to get away with seemed harmless, it was wrong for me to put myself in situations that jeopardized my faith and compromised my beliefs. There is never an excuse for sin. Obedience to God is always the greater necessity. As we follow Jesus, we must be able to discern what to think, what to say, and what to do based on the objective truth that God is sovereign. That is where The Holy Spirit comes in.

Wherever God's activities are, therein lies His spirit. His spirit was present and active during the creation of time, space, the world, and everything in it.

> *In the beginning, God created the heavens and the earth. . . . And **the Spirit of God** was hovering over the face of the waters.*
>
> —Gen. 1:1–2

As for the creation of human beings, God said,

> **Let us make man in our image, after our likeness.**
>
> —Gen. 1:26

The word *us* refers to the triune order: Father, Son, and, indeed, the Holy Spirit. These three persons who make up one entity are represented here on earth by your mind, your body, and your soul—wonderful, powerful connections, with which come tremendous and weighty responsibility. They enable us to see things from God's perspective, to love Jesus while learning His ways, and to live by the Holy Spirit's strength and support.

Today, we need the Holy Spirit for our spiritual health and our physical fitness. He helps us walk in all the ways of Jesus with full confidence as it pertains to His will for our temporary bodies and the restoration of our souls. This promised spirit gives us citizenship into heaven along with divine power to overcome the misery and deprivation of death, our greatest curse. It is a power that only believers in Jesus can receive and that no one can offer besides God.

Religions, cults, and various sects worldwide would beg to differ with this power of the Holy Spirit in our lives. That is why, when pursuing spiritual health and fitness, we must be mindful of spirits that are not from God. Those doctrines advertise a different way to live and, most often, a different afterlife. When I conducted research on other belief systems, the one that was most concerning was actually the fixed order of non-belief found in atheism.

Atheists do not acknowledge the existence of God the creator, Jesus the savior, or the Holy Spirit, our helper. According to atheist belief, there is no afterlife; we all simply cease to exist. One thing Christians and atheists agree on is that all bodies end up in the ground or cremated one day. Yes, there will be a day for all of us when personal training, aerobics, conditioning, and healthy habits will matter no more. So don't take care of your body in hopes of living as long as possible. Instead, nurture your body as a demonstration of stewardship and gratefulness to Him who gave you your body.

Paul the apostle wrote:

So, whether you eat or drink, or whatever you do, do all to the glory of God.

—1 Cor. 10:31

That is what it's all about. We do everything for God's glory. When we allow the Holy Spirit to come into our lives, we enter into a redeemed state that allows us to glorify God with our bodies. We are then affected spiritually toward salvation and physically toward good health. By allowing God's word to define our purpose through faith, we find our identity in the teachings of Jesus who perfectly glorified God in all He did.

By listening to Jesus, we open our ears to the Holy Spirit's voice and receive instruction on how we should then live. Giving God authority over our bodies so He can govern how we diet and exercise is a big part of doing "all to the glory of God." While we're in these bodies, we allow God's spirit into our hearts, minds, and souls so He can teach us to eat faithfully, drink appropriately, think positively, and act biblically.

You see, God created us to remain in constant communication with Him, to receive truth and attain wisdom and guidance. Living holistically by the Holy Spirit helps us cultivate a relationship with God so we can run to Him for counsel in all things. Jesus, who was full of the Holy Spirit (Luke 4:1), perfectly embraced this fellowship in every aspect to achieve what only He and God and the power of the Holy Spirit could achieve—victory over evil and iniquity. Within the perfect will and sovereign plan of God, the Holy Spirit is ever flowing as protector, instructor, and helper.

We Must Not Reject His Protection

We ought to be dependent on the Holy Spirit who provides refuge and has the power to safeguard us from spiritual and physical attacks. Throughout my history, I've seen the Holy Spirit do the unthinkable, making Him a monumental factor in providing strength for God's work. However, I still ignored Him, erring and egotistically going astray. It's as if I'd been coerced into accepting, based on others' success, that self-reliance is somehow superior to heavenly succor from the hand that created the entire cosmos. That tended to shift my focus from living a life that was centered on God to one that was self-serving. It then became easy to allow things like money and sex to be the apple of my eye. The Holy Spirit is meant to guard us against this mindset so we don't wander down a path of self-indulgence. Unrestrained gratification of our own spiritual and physical appetites equals bred-in-the-bone deterioration of our health and fitness.

In the book of Judges, chapters 13 through 16, is the story of Samson, who was once ruler over Israel, chosen by God to free His people from Philistine oppression. In the telling of Samson's life, we see this combination of divine intervention versus masculine mishap. It is a prime example of God's desire to protect and man's proneness to defect. Starting with the introduction to Samson's parents, who are God-fearing, humble people, the angel of the Lord appears to them with news of an upcoming physical miracle.

> *Behold, you are barren and have not borne children, but you shall conceive and bear a son. **Therefore be careful and drink no wine or strong drink, and eat nothing unclean**. . . . No razor shall come upon his head, for the child shall be a Nazirite to God from the womb, and he shall begin to save Israel from the hand of the Philistines.*
>
> —Judges 13:3–5

Samson was to be set apart for God's work and purposes. As such, there were physical requirements he and his parents needed to abide by. After he was born, God blessed Samson and began to impel him in the ways of strength, honor, service, and battle. As a grown man, though, Samson got too big for his britches, cocky even. He opted to start making decisions on his own in an unwise manner. Regardless of what his calling was, he took it upon himself to ignore the stirring in him that God began when He set him apart.

Samson's first mistake was rebelling against his parents' wishes and condoning what was wrong in the sight of God.

> *I saw one of the daughters of the Philistines at Timnah.* ***Now get her for me as my wife.... Get her for me for she is right in my eyes.***
> —Judges 14:2–3

On the way to make arrangements with his soon-to-be fiancée, Samson encountered a young lion in one of the vineyards. God, seeking to protect Samson, empowered him with His Holy Spirit. God preserved Samson's life and health with bold courage and extraordinary strength.

> *And behold, a young lion came toward him roaring. Then* ***the Spirit of the Lord rushed upon him, and although he had nothing in his hand, he tore the lion in pieces*** *as one tears a young goat.*
> —Judges 14:5–6

Sometime later, Samson returned to the dead animal and saw that a swarm of bees had produced honey inside of it. Going against God's law, he not only touched and ate something unclean, but he also gave some of the honey to his parents to eat, deceiving them by not telling them he got it from the defiled carcass of a lion. What we see happening resembles the behavior of a man believing the lie that what feels right for his body is more important than what God sees fit for the body.

For Samson, it didn't stop there. Succumbed to selfish gain, he made a bet he thought he could easily win. When it backfired on him, God had to protect him once again from trouble over a gambling debt.

> *And the Spirit of the LORD rushed upon him, and he went down to Ashkelon and struck down thirty men of the town and took their spoil and gave the garments to those who had told the riddle. In hot anger he went back to his father's house.*
>
> —Judges 14:19

Although God was gracious enough to empower Samson by the Holy Spirit with strength and skill, Samson was definitely abusing his power. His actions were filling him with sinful rage and impure hostility. He was stuck in a bitter and vengeful state that only added fuel to the fire in the war between Israel and Philistia.

> *So Samson went and caught 300 foxes and took torches. And he turned them tail to tail and put a torch between each pair of tails. And when he had set fire to the torches, he let the foxes go into the standing grain of the Philistines and set fire to the stacked grain and the standing grain, as well as the olive orchards. . . . And he said to them, **"As they did to me, so I have done to them."***
>
> —Judges 15:4–5, 11

This act of retaliation set off a chain reaction that provoked anger in the hearts of the men whose food supplies were ruined. Part of the blame ended up falling on Samson's wife and father-in-law.

Although they had nothing to do with the fires, the Philistines had them burned to death.

We Must Not Get Caught Up in Ourselves

What's interesting at this point in the story is that there hadn't been any dialogue between God and Samson. It helps us conclude that these actions most likely weren't sanctioned by God and that Samson was merely responding to how he felt in the moment. Samson was set apart to be a spiritual leader, yet we haven't heard him pray, encourage, or offer anything up to God. He doesn't seem to have any interest in saving Israel from the Philistines. His life has been all about him, even though God has been by his side since birth.

In the next part of the story, Samson was restrained and handed over to his enemies, and still God protected him.

> *Then the Spirit of the LORD rushed upon him, and the ropes that were on his arms became as flax that has caught fire, and his bonds melted off his hands. And he found a fresh jawbone of a donkey, and put out his hand and took it, and with it he struck 1,000 men.*
>
> —Judges 15:14–15

You would think that after this miraculous display of divine rescue by the Holy Spirit, Samson would raise his hands to the sky and lift his eyes up to heaven to thank and praise God for protecting him. Well, he didn't. Instead, he seized the opportunity to draw attention to himself.

> *And Samson said, "With the jawbone of a donkey, heaps upon heaps . . . have I struck down a thousand men."*
>
> —Judges 15:16

Then, after he finished bragging about himself, he complained to God about how thirsty he was, as if God is some water boy.

> *"You have granted this great salvation by the hand of your servant, and shall I now die of thirst and fall into the hands of the uncircumcised?" And God split open the hollow place that is at Lehi, and water came out from it. And when he drank, his spirit returned, and he revived.*
>
> —Judges 15:18–19

This is the testimony of a man obsessed with meeting his own needs, and of God the father faithfully meeting His child's spiritual and physical needs. But Samson continued to grow arrogant and became immoral. He wanted the power of the Holy Spirit without the incumbency of bearing the image of God as a holy man to the people. He enjoyed the high stature and the fame. He glorified himself on his own grandstand in his winning and triumph, becoming blind to the fact that God was his upper hand. The Holy Spirit's surety eventually left Samson feeble and exposed due to his apostasy and unruly ways. It was then that his life took a turn for the worse and sank into a downward spiral.

> *"But he did not know that **the LORD had left him**. And the Philistines seized him and gouged out his eyes . . . and bound him with bronze shackles. And he ground at the mill in the prison.*
>
> —Judges 16:20–21

This is the type of outcome for people who neglect the righteous spirit of God for the false apparition of themselves. This is the kind of misery I was in when I rejected the spiritual and physical requirements God wanted me to keep. When I resisted God in the body, it became difficult for me to be empowered by the Holy Spirit and live under His protection.

For Samson, it took physical blindness to get him to see his spiritual blindness. Solitary confinement helped him realize what a fool he'd been. The slave labor he was now forced to perform surely convicted him of his many shortcomings, including the constant abuse of the Holy Spirit's power. He eventually pleaded to God for help. In his final prayer to God, he asked for justice.

> O LORD God, please remember me and please strengthen me only this once, O God, that I may be avenged on the Philistines for my two eyes. . . . Let me die with the Philistines.
>
> —Judges 16:28–30

Because of his humility and his willingness to finally submit to God and trust in the power of the Holy Spirit, by faith, Samson was empowered one final time so the people of Israel could be delivered from their enemy's hands and God's mission could be completed. Samson died a hero, but it's sad that his life had to end in tragedy. Some might say he chose to learn the hard way, which was, unfortunately, down a path of collateral damage and dismay.

> Then he bowed with all his strength, and the house fell upon the lords and upon all the people who were in it. So the dead whom he killed at his death were more than those whom he had killed during his life.
>
> —Judges 16:30

Samson goes down in history as a man of brave faith whom God made strong out of weakness. But because we know the character of God, we can be sure the story would have been different if Samson hadn't been reluctant to obey God or if he hadn't ignored the training of God's spirit.

Let the Holy Spirit Instruct Your Body

Today, there are millions of men and women whose pursuit of health and fitness resembles Samson's former character. A lot of weight rooms are filling up with men gawking at women, women seducing men, concerned about what their bodies can do for themselves rather than their creator. They walk around spiritually blind, philandering with whomever they choose, neglecting God's authority in their lives. I can say so because I've kept company with such women and men. I was even one of them.

All we seemed to care about was looking good and getting laid. For me, every visit to the gym was to feed my ego, to build my self-esteem and self-worth, to look better naked. It's disgusting how I only seemed to work out when all the hot girls were there so I could feast my eyes on their revealing sports bras and skimpy yoga pants. It is in every single one of those moments that I subconsciously rejected the safekeeping of the Holy Spirit.

The measure of a man is not his love life, his biceps, or his paycheck. The measure of a woman is not her sex appeal, her petite bikini body, or hard-earned independence. Masculinity and femininity are weighed upon the strength and fruit of the Holy Spirit: love and faithfulness, self-control and dignity, teachability, and humility. We don't make a difference in the world by how much money and fame we possess. We better the world by being men and women who talk to God through prayer, who seek to know Him more by reading His Word, and who ask Him questions with a heart that truly seeks His advice. Followers of Jesus, people of character, people of bravery, are the people the Holy Spirit literally sets apart and empowers to do God's work.

While they were worshiping the Lord and fasting, the Holy Spirit said, "Set apart for me Barnabas and Saul for the work to which I have called them."

—Acts 13:2

We need the Holy Spirit's instruction in everything. Modern people have become no stranger to unhealthy filth, vanity, and bodily greed. Doesn't it seem that we've become a people of hyperconsumption and cravings? From Margarita Monday to Black Friday, from professional football on Sunday to college ball on Saturday. Let's not forget Taco Tuesday and the famous Hump Day. We're just following the crowd and the excitement. Soon we'll have a day for everything delectable—National Pancake Day, National Fried Chicken Day, National Doughnut Day, National Pizza Day. Where are our priorities when it comes to how we treat our bodies?

Be Mission-Minded and Mission-Bodied

Imagine what we could do if we redirected the billions of dollars we eat to satisfy the munchies. What could we do with the billions of dollars wasted on getting wasted? Together, we could probably end poverty and hunger. Cure cancer maybe? How about we rescue a third-world country by giving up our first-world tendencies? Wouldn't that be awesome? The people of God are capable of doing that through the power of the Holy Spirit.

The part of the world that's starving needs to be fed the fortified love of Jesus spiritually and physically. As a former couch potato and videogamer, I knew society wouldn't be impacted or inspired by me unless I became a man who fears God, ready to run the race of faith and finish strong. I knew my community would never benefit if I stood in front of a mirror all day taking selfies. Our communities need people filled with the spirit who can stand on the front lines of churches, doing the heavy lifting at outreaches both locally and globally. The world needs the hands and feet of Jesus along with the arms and legs of His people.

Jesus Christ lived on a mission, and so must we. If He needed the power of the Holy Spirit, how much more do we? The Holy Spirit's counsel and advice apply 24 hours a day, seven days a week. We must take it, or we will be taken. God has not spared anything from us—not His son, not His spirit—all of Him is at our disposal. Let's give God exclusive rights to our thoughts, our emotions, all parts of our body, and every component of our soul.

For too many years, I was dependent upon "me time" and relaxation. That was a tough place to be as a Christian. Living for God was exhausting when things weren't going my way or turning out the way I expected. Many times I'd leave God at the front door of a local brewery while I drowned my stress in a bucket of ice-cold beers. At the gym, I would stuff God into a gym bag and leave Him in a locker room while I sweated out my frustration. We should never want to take a break from God. He's the one who rejuvenates and recharges us.

The Holy Spirit is our fuel as well. He is our body pump. And He never takes a break from us. There's never a moment when He needs a vacation or an escape from working in us. Every time I felt as if He wasn't there to help me, I was always the one who had distanced myself from Him. I was always the one who was partial to Him. In fact, it's only when I ignore the Holy Spirit that I commit sin and wrongdoing. He has cautioned every one of us about crimes against God. Those same crimes can be committed against our own bodies in a way that dishonors Him, like gluttony and sloth. We must keep our bodies strong so we can use our strength to serve God.

Let the Holy Spirit Help Your Body

What we see played out in the Bible, in both the Old and New Testaments, is God the father, Jesus the son, and the Holy Spirit enduring the flaws and imperfections of humankind, suffering long for the sake of righteousness and glory. God's people have a history of abusing their bodies in every way, even inventing new ways to mishandle their health, affecting the wellness of others in the process.

But we see God's faithfulness in the provision of physical miracles and marvelous teaching for the body and soul. His people are filled with awe and good health at the sound of divine revelation and the sight of His strength in non-stop action during times of revival and peace, but also through war, hardship, and adversity.

> *Behold, God is my helper; the Lord is the upholder of my life.*
>
> —Ps. 54:4

God is our ultimate source for liveliness. Even in His own silence He speaks volumes over all the noisy chaos that burdens and distracts us. Even by His delay, He demonstrates fitting love and care. Even His anger and wrath reveal protection for strength and deliverance from weakness. Nothing can minimize the great lengths He has gone to for His people. His toil on our behalf is why we exalt Him as undeniable, and then His unyielding courage comes to us by the power of His spirit.

We need the Holy Spirit's help, and we need it desperately. Although life can effectuate vast progressive movement toward enlightenment and understanding, it is also filled with enigmatic complexities. Whenever we align our life with the Spirit, we reap the benefits He freely gives us, both spiritually and physically. He provides perfect clarity for the body and the mind, He increases our enthusiasm and our energy, and He overcomes all mental and physical strain.

Jesus Was Empowered by the Spirit

The night before Jesus's death was surely fraught with anguish and despair. It was characterized by the troubled soul of Jesus who knew His cross was at hand and by the troubled hearts of His disciples who were about to lose their father figure and mentor, their brother and peerless companion. Jesus would soon be betrayed and forsaken. Those closest to Him would soon be sheep without a shepherd. So knowing that His departure would devastate them, Jesus made a promise in their time of need. He left them with peace and hope, guaranteeing the Holy Spirit would be sent down from God, to not only be with them, but to be in them.

> *But the Helper, the Holy Spirit, whom the Father will send in my name, he will teach you all things and bring to your remembrance all that I have said to you.*
>
> —John 14:26

The ministry of Jesus opened entirely with the Holy Spirit. He was what made Jesus rock solid in His body and unbreakable in His mind. Jesus's empowerment began with the Spirit descending on Him at baptism, was completed by the Spirit at the cross, and was passed on through the Spirit to His disciples.

> *And when he had said this, he breathed on them and said to them, "Receive the Holy Spirit."*
>
> —John 20:22

His purpose would be to guide them spiritually in the ways of the Shepherd: love, righteousness, and truth. His voice would serve as a conscious reminder of Christ, their Mediator.

Look carefully then how you walk, not as unwise but as wise, making the best use of the time, because the days are evil. Therefore do not be foolish, but understand what the will of the LORD is. And do not get drunk with wine ... but be filled with the Spirit ... giving thanks always and for everything to God the Father in the name of our LORD Jesus Christ.
—Eph. 5:15–20

Jesus, with the help of the Holy Spirit, was able to inspire people and imprint on them power for strength and endurance, physically and spiritually. That was something Samson failed to do, and that's a shame. While we remember Samson as a hero, let us never forget the righteous pain and godly grief that can be inflicted upon the Holy Spirit.

By the mighty breath of Jesus, let us be faithful emissaries of this great power, never exploiting it, so we are constantly fueled with the spirit of God and never falter by the spirit of selfishness. Samson nearly destroyed the work of God, wasting time on things that were meaningless. May we never seek to improve our minds or our bodies by vainly and selfishly empowering our flesh, but by the unmatchable strength of the Holy Spirit.

Be Humbled by the Holy Spirit

We are accompanied by His presence so we don't make the mistake of trying to figure out life on our own. When it was time for me to break the cycle of living in my own sinew and puissance, I was looking everywhere else and to everyone else for empowerment. Even as it was so easy for me to be lazy or run to all my vices, there was abundant mercy made available in the virtue of the cross. So the proper response for me was to fall down on my knees and pray. I asked the Holy Spirit to restore me with His strength, and God poured out His grace on me. It was then that the Spirit reminded me to live in light of what Jesus accomplished for us.

> *Blessed be the God and Father of our Lord Jesus Christ! According to his great mercy, he has caused us to be born again to a living hope through the resurrection of Jesus Christ from the dead, to an inheritance that is imperishable, undefiled, and unfading, kept in heaven for you, who by God's power are being guarded through faith for a salvation ready to be revealed in the last time.*
>
> —1 Pet. 1:3–5

As we live life, our thoughts, our decisions, and our actions should begin with the undeniable fact and amazing truth that God exists in power outside of time and space. He is not restricted to a clock or a calendar nor weakened by heat or chill. God is not subject to day or night, and there is no beginning or end with Him. He is forever strong, and in that strength, He has saved us a spot in eternity with Him. God makes His decisions in light of eternity and empowers us with His Holy Spirit to do the same.

If we are going to make it a habit to pray, then let's pray in the direction and power of the Holy Spirit. If we are going to ask God for things such as a good job, good health, or a better body, then once He gives it to us, we should work dutifully, pursuing the eternal fruits of the Spirit—integrity, sobriety, and dignity.

We should walk with Him and not in opposition to Him so that when we do spiritual things such as bless a meal by saying grace, thankful to God for our food, we can partake of it free from gluttony and void of any ungodliness. Having this perception equips our bodies to be faithful stewards and more effective ministers in all seasons, at all ages, and under all conditions.

CHAPTER 4

Nothing without Love

Some think love is that warm fuzzy feeling you get when snuggled up with a significant other. Some think love is that satisfying savory goodness that hits your lips when you drink a beer or that sensation on your tongue when you bite into a juicy cheeseburger or a hot slice of pizza. Some believe all you need is love, while others will tell you love is a battlefield and a mere secondhand emotion. People say love hurts or love stinks, yet so many of us would do anything for love. Some of us are addicted to love and so crazy in love. But really, what is love?

Love Defined and Displayed

Love is the ultimate motive for living well, the most powerful source for health and the most fundamental component for fitness. Love is strong and enduring. It's priceless and timeless. It has the power to conquer all things and to make all things new. Since God is who He is, it's only fair that our definition of love derives from Him. God is also strong and enduring, priceless and timeless. Love originates from God because God is love (1 John 4:8). He has singlehandedly conquered our sin and renewed our minds. He captivates the hearts of those who believe in Him, to put love in them through the humble and selfless servant, Jesus.

When Jesus knew that his hour had come to depart out of this world to the Father, having loved his own who were in the world, he loved them to the end. Jesus, knowing that the Father had given all things into his hands, and that he had come from God and was going back to God, rose from supper.... Then He poured water into a basin and began to wash the disciples' feet.

—John 13:1, 2–5

On Jesus's final night on earth at His last meal with His disciples, He performed a lower-class duty, one of the most dirty, menial tasks—washing their feet. Knowing full well the great tragedy that was soon approaching and who would be responsible for His betrayal and murder, He continued firmly according to God's plan without complaint. Even as He was master and lord to them, He lovingly cleansed them. Even in their incompetence, even with all their mistakes, infractions, and idiosyncrasies, Jesus had one mission, a call to sacrificial love. This demonstration of humility and devotion of service to them reveals His unadulterated passion for His people.

Love Discarded and Despised

Biblical history is filled with beautiful demonstrations of the love of Jesus. However, modern history shows us that the world has become tone-deaf to the harmony of the gospel. Instead of heeding the call to God's love, the world has hearkened to a call for superiority, provocation, and defense. But this attitude is nothing new to humanity. Paul the apostle tells us that the way of lovelessness has always existed in the hearts of humankind.

As it is written: "None is righteous, no, not one; no one understands; no one seeks for God. All have turned aside; together they have become worthless; no one does good, not even one. Their throat is an open grave; they use their tongues to deceive. The venom of asps is under their lips. Their mouth is full of curses and bitterness. Their feet are swift to shed blood; in their paths are ruin and misery, and the way of peace they have not known. There is no fear of God before their eyes."

—Rom. 3:10–18

In 1941, the world was at war. The Nazis were murdering hundreds of thousands of Jews by German firing squads, with poisonous gas, and even by burying them alive. German concentration camps were filled with the sound of mothers wailing as families were being torn apart and destroyed. Wives were being made into widows as their husbands' resistance was short-lived. Children could only watch as their parents were killed right before their own eyes. Things worsened when the Japanese launched a surprise attack on American soil. Pearl Harbor's battleships were demolished by air strikes, torpedoes, and kamikaze pilots. Thousands of US military servicemen and women lost their lives within a matter of just a couple of hours, leaving a world superpower shocked and shaken, forcing a national call to fight back.

Thirty years later, in 1971, John Lennon was sitting at his Steinway piano at his estate in England. With a misguided, yet heavy heart he wrote a song called "Imagine," inspired by his wife's poems and a Christian prayer book. In the melody, you can hear he's tired and weary, concerned for his fellow man. He was saddened by all the hate that had spread across the nations, and the divisiveness got to him. He wrote thinking of the soldiers in Vietnam that died every day by the hundreds, who were caught up in a war he didn't believe would bring peace. He also took issue with how the rich seemed to neglect the poor, sickened by the elite's materialism. The idea of heaven and hell bothered him. He was fed up with the condemning judgmental ways of religious fanatics and was left wondering why we were unable to share the earth together. His voice would convey a global message of revolution and a call to action.

Another 30 years went by, and in 2001, terrorists hijacked airplanes from major airlines and used them to blow up buildings in New York. This erupted into widespread panic, chaos, and awakening in the city that never sleeps. The world watched in horror as smoke and flames filled the sky. Firefighters and policemen were diligent in evacuating the city to try to minimize the number of injuries and death. Debris and ashes fell everywhere around the Twin Towers along with a number of human beings who plummeted to their deaths. While the government scrambled to figure out who or what was responsible, you can be sure this mayhem was brewing into a major call to retaliation.

Love Begins with God

Think about what life is like today. What seems to be modern society's call? Jews are still being persecuted. Ties are closer between the United States and some foreign countries but worse with others. Our nation still suffers from racism and disunity, and the war on terror continues. Some of us, along with those people of high power, position, and reputation through all those events, gave rise to the image of a world without God. Humans have missed the truth that no matter how many battles they win or how many songs they write or how much terror they cause, they can never create a world of peace and unity without the love of the Lord.

What do you think life will be like in 2031? What will the call be then? Will there be a call to protest? A call to boycott? Who can know? Will there be a call to co-exist? A call to battle?

No one can really be sure. But, we *can* know that regardless of how many burdensome conflicts arise, how depressing the days become, or how great the trial or tribulation, there will always be a definite call to love.

When I look at my past, I can identify with the unhealthy hate and corruption that destroys hearts and minds. They also caused me to neglect God, my first love, my one truest love. By His grace, I have learned that without love, we cannot be like Christ. Jesus didn't come into the world to annihilate people or commit genocide for power and sovereign rule. He didn't come to protest the government or start anti-war campaigns for peace. He wasn't here to terrorize with bombs and weapons of mass destruction. He came to begin the unstoppable force of the body of Christ called the church. To do that, He had one job: die in our place because of our sin to deliver us from wrath.

For even the Son of Man came not to be served but to serve, and to give his life as a ransom for many.

—Mark 10:45

This charge He received from God, His father, and He carried out His objective through the strength and power of the Holy Spirit. This divine operation wasn't motivated by racial supremacy or vengeful hatred; it was motivated by everlasting love. Love is the main ingredient for mind renewal, soul conversion, and lifelong body transformation. Its power existed long before you, me, and the entire human race. God's love has been around forever, and it has never failed; it will never die, and it will overcome anything that tries to stop it.

Think back on the creation of the world in the first chapter of Genesis in the Bible. Within the first few verses, we read that God gave us two essentials that make life possible on earth: water and light. Next, He gave us fish, dry land for fruits and vegetables, and then lamb, goats, cows, turkeys, and chickens. After that, Adam and Eve were created to be together, representing the first couple, and God initiated the opportunity for billions upon billions of people to have a chance at life. God took the nothingness of what we would never be and turned it into the fullness of what we now live and breathe, even though it would require the future sacrifice of His son on the cross. That is love!

Everything God provides for us is exactly what we'd expect from a loving father. He forged for us food, care, and shelter, but He didn't stop there. God blessed us with ability—the ability to work, to be led by Him, and to lead others. He gave us the ability to procreate, to build, and invent. God blessed us with desire—the desire to love and thrive, the desire for joy and pleasure, celebration, and triumph, the desire to learn and share, inform and pass on.

This is my commandment, that you love one another as I have loved you. Greater love has no one than this, that someone lay down his life for his friends. You are my friends if you do what I command you.
—John 15:12–14

You see, we shouldn't waste time trying to imagine there's no heaven or no God, because the original source of love flows from Him and is Him. And if you've ever felt true love, whether through relationships, your career, or your hobbies, I believe you have felt the very presence of God Himself. To imagine away God would be to imagine away all things that pertain to love and define love. God is love, Jesus Christ is our peace, and the unbreakable bond that unites every believer as family is the Holy Spirit.

We Are Called to Love Our Bodies

The call to love is a call that includes bodily integrity. Jesus said that if we are truly His followers, we will abide in His love by keeping His commandments. If we are truly Christians, we must be men and women of biblical honesty and blamelessness. The more veracious our hearts and minds, the more joy and health are divinely transferred to us in full. Jesus said this is like being good trees that bear good fruit. He often referred to Himself as living water and the light of the world, which are both necessary for growth and enrichment.

> *Either make the tree good and its fruit good, or make the tree bad and its fruit bad, for the tree is known by its fruit.*
>
> —Matt. 12:33

Too often, I sold myself short of the perfect joy and happiness God makes available. I don't think I ever actually wanted to be a bad tree bearing bad fruit, but what I did want was something much worse: to have the appearance of good fruit without taking on the responsibility of being a good tree. Here's another way to put it. I wanted to reap the benefits of the light while still keeping secrets in the dark.

On some levels, I can relate to professional and college athletes who have been caught swindling their way to championships and record-breaking success. I'm sure if I had been in their shoes, I would have found ways to cheat, too. But it's still sad to watch some of our favorite sports heroes plague themselves with scandals because of doping for dishonest gain. I believe that being motivated by the love of God gives us the power to avoid such unfortunate outcomes.

When we love our bodies the way God loves our bodies, we can avoid lies and deception. Perfect love puts an end to our being disqualified or stripped of our gold crowns spiritually and physically.

Only the love of God enables us to truly be the best and at the top of our game. It prevents the worst from coming out in the end. It shines brighter than any other global spotlight and extends our prime into eternity.

Thank God for His "scandal" of grace. Thank God that His call to unconditional love can mend damaged reputations so we can sprint after His ways of wisdom and walk with transparency.

> *Whoever walks in integrity walks securely, but he who makes his ways crooked will be found out. The mouth of the righteous is a fountain of life, but the mouth of the wicked conceals violence. Hatred stirs up strife, but* **love** *covers all offenses.*
>
> —Prov. 10:9, 11–12

Every day, the call to integrity is ignored on the grounds that vainglory and selfish enterprise take precedence over sound mind, body, and soul. But that doesn't just happen in the big leagues. It starts locally in our schools and recreation centers. It creeps into big corporate fitness clubs and mom-and-pop gyms with small-time people just like you and me. Many are the temptations along the journey to health and fitness, but the greatest combatant is love.

Love stops corruption and deterioration of health on all levels. Only love can stop a pregnant mom from drinking, smoking, and using drugs. Only love can enable an overweight dad to play more softball with his daughter and more basketball with his son. Love can help parents decide to discontinue the processed foods train that is railroading our kids into obesity. Love is strong enough to carry the heavy burden of dieting and exercise to fight diseases that are killing people every single day. Love brings us out of hiding from the shame of being unhealthy and out of shape.

I remember when my health and my body were too much of a private matter that I had become an easy target for bearing bad fruit in the dark. My motivation behind a noticeable physique was a self-centered preventative measure for insecurity and embarrassment. Self-centered fear of getting fat and overweight led to a battle with bulimia that did more harm than good. The lack of godly fear caused me to eat whatever I wanted at the neglect of well-being, leaving me to resort to the unhealthy practice of making myself throw up, going on crash diets, and starving myself.

We Are Called to Control Our Impulses

Sometimes the struggle isn't to stay thin but to get thick. Craving for increased muscle mass had me breaking the law to use non-prescribed steroids and other performance-enhancing drugs. Substance abusers in every form serve as a misrepresentation of what God created us to be. Jesus never lied to get His way and never cheated to get ahead. We must allow His incorruptible Holy Spirit to inspire our physique by guiding our hearts and appetites. Trust in Heaven's champion who has immeasurable strength, countless riches, and victory that never ends.

The call to love is a call to self-control (Titus 2:1–15). Some people think the greatest human strength is willpower. But willpower without conviction can most certainly be dangerous. As we've seen and heard, it can turn male and female competitors into criminals greedy for more home runs, gold medals, and race titles. Willpower without truth can convince a liar to keep on lying, to cover up and deceive. Willpower without Jesus's love can cause self-absorption, and without God's love, it can cause self-destruction. The devil and his wreckage on earth is the prime example of willpower gone wrong.

In Genesis chapter 2, before the devil's scheme unfolds, we get a glimpse of Adam's wholesome character and how he represented

God well. God had lovingly set everything up for human beings, the world at their feet, beginning with a paradise of bliss and the perfect place for Adam and Eve to raise a family. Adam never complained about anything. He gladly took on work and responsibility. There was a perfect balance that existed in everything, including Adam's physical features and attributes. Adam never overate or gorged, and he was never gluttonous. He cared for his body, his muscles, his organs, and his senses in the same way he cared for the grounds in the perfect Garden of Eden.

He understood very well that God was in charge, and he willingly obeyed in submission. When Eve showed up in her perfect naked body, it's worth noting that Adam didn't lust after her. He didn't objectify her, worship her, or seek to take advantage of her. He had no temptation to masturbate, abuse her sexually, or cause any type of physical anguish or disorder. Instead, he delighted in her, knowing full well this beautiful and physically fit woman was God's gift to him.

He continued in his upright masculinity by loving her, naming her, leading her, nourishing her, and sharing all his knowledge with her about God's will and God's commands. It wasn't until the devil showed up in Genesis chapter 3 that everything went awry. Although psychotic and delusional, the devil was slippery enough to ensnare Eve, tricking her into disobeying God.

Her willpower was bent by his swagger and sway, revealing her lack of self-constraint and a desire for unrestrained gratification. In that moment, Eve was so fixed on herself that she neglected her call to be an undaunted helper fit for Adam, who was also at fault since he did nothing to stop her, contributing to this unthinkable act. For the first time, love was distorted, tainted, and confused. Adam and Eve felt guilt and shame, a condition that caused them to run and hide from God.

God Commands Love for Our Good

Too many of us today have been hurt by a lack of self-control and the effects of distorted love. We are running and hiding from God when we should be pursuing Him in all things daily. Every waking moment, God desires to commune with us. He wants to be involved in what we eat for breakfast, how we dress, how we spend our time. As the knower of all things with unlimited understanding and infinite power, God is there to guide us in our decisions on the road, at work, at the gym, in our relationships, and as we work toward our goals.

We spend a lot of time searching for the right answers, peace of mind, love, and happiness, and all the while, God is available to provide them and even more. God's word contains the solutions for life's problems and the tools to overcome adversity. His word is probably sitting on a book shelf not far from you. The words of Jesus call out to us from it to give us insight. Open your heart and be restored to God spiritually and physically through the love of Jesus, who said this:

> *If you love me, you will keep my commandments . . . If anyone loves me,*
> *he will keep my word, and my Father will love him, and we will come*
> *to him and make our home with him.*
>
> —John 14:15, 23

What better way for us to get in shape and stay in shape than to have almighty God come to us and make His home with us. Jesus speaks in many distinct ways through His word so we must always be listening. He can speak through world history, through American history, through a local community, through weird spiritual coworkers, and even through those Bible-thumping friends of ours. Chances are that God has put people in our lives who have a love for spiritual and physical fitness through their faith. Their witness and testimony serve as a way to get our attention and draw us near to God.

If we allow ourselves to be distracted by self-interest, we could miss valuable counsel on how to love our bodies and have a love for fitness. If, in those opportunities to listen for what's best, we hear only what we want to hear, we might miss out on what could be healthy training and instruction. God intends to release us from the bondage of this world by teaching us to cut ties with impulsive behaviors that subtly induce self-absorption.

Rejecting the call to self-control thrusted me into bad eating habits and alcoholism. As a former non-believer, I used to rack my brain trying to figure out life on my own, obsessed with self-reliance and desperate to be self-sufficient. But I had put my trust in dirty needles, black-market pills, one-night stands, money, and comfort food. God's love was the invaluable key that set me free from all that so I could set in motion my own personal faith-infused fitness. Today, His love encourages me to live wholeheartedly by the Holy Spirit who guards my blind side from opposing attacks and potentially harmful tendencies (Gal. 5:16).

We Fight for Love Together

None of us is alone in this battle. Together, we should be side-by-side, running the good race, where at the finish line, Jesus promises a crown of endurance, a reward that can never be stripped away.

> *I have fought the good fight, I have finished the race, I have kept the faith. . . . There is laid up for me the crown of righteousness, which the* LORD *. . . will give to me on that day, and not to me only but also to all who have loved his appearing.*
>
> —2 Tim. 4:7–8

The call to love is a call to serve others (Lev. 19:17–18). From Genesis to Revelation is the story of God's outward demonstration of self-giving love toward a people of inward focus. In this story, we learn the two main components of living a life of the fullest health and purest fitness—to love the Lord your God with all your heart, mind, soul, and strength, and love your neighbor as yourself (Mark 12:29–31). Everything we do—or don't do—must stem from these two commandments. Why? Because everything God does and doesn't do is out of love for His son, His spirit, His kingdom, and His people.

What does it mean to love God with all that we are? It means that every part of us belongs to Him and is for Him. Our body is His, so if we love Him, we will nourish it, cherish it, and protect it in every way. That means digesting only what is good for the heart and thinking about only what is good for the mind. Embracing only what is good for the soul enables us to take part in what is best for our strength. If we love God with our entire being, He receives glory and honor from all that we are.

Let's say there are two Christian guys—Fred and Charlie—living next door to each other. Fred spends his Saturdays in the hot sun feeding the homeless, while Charlie lounges in his bedroom drinking wildly and stuffing his face with food. Which one brought more glory and honor to God that day? Suppose on Sundays they both go to church. Fred arrives early to help set up and greet others as they walk in, while Charlie shows up late, hung over, and sits in the back where it's easier to doze off. Which one better represents the heart and soul of Jesus? On Mondays, they both go to the gym. Fred silently prays for an opportunity to evangelize someone, while Charlie secretly plots to have sex with the blonde bombshell in the skin-tight shorts. Which of them seems to be more in step with the Holy Spirit?

Loving God with all that we are makes us even more fit to love and serve others. Sure, Fred seems like a solid Christian, seeking after God physically and spiritually. But it sounds like he needs to reach out to Charlie as soon as possible. What good is it for Fred to flourish in Christ while his neighbor backslides? This story reminds me that Jesus has put the light of the world in me. My light is no good to anyone if I keep it in the dark. Answering the call to love means looking out for others, not just myself. If God's love is impacting my health for the good, I should want to impact others through His love for their good.

Iron sharpens iron, and one man sharpens another.

—Prov. 27:17

God's Love Makes Us Stronger

The love of God is contagious, as is His strength and the power of His Holy Spirit. We have the potential and privilege to impart many virtues through His love, including courage, energy, dexterity, and persistence. All these are essential for faith, spiritually and physically. They prevent us from being sloppy servants. They bar us from getting lazy and becoming mere spectators that sit back and just let life happen to us. They keep us sharp and on our toes. This state of all-around fitness better equips us for the call to ministry at any given moment, from the crack of dawn through all hours of the night. It supplies us with an arsenal of edifying words for Bible studies, debates, and the call to defend the gospel.

Him we proclaim, warning everyone and teaching everyone with all wisdom, that we may present everyone mature in Christ. For this I toil, struggling with all his energy that he powerfully works within me.

—Col. 1:28

We already know that love spiritually improves marriages, relationships, and people's drive for life and success. But physically, love can make more able-bodied parents and more effective ministers and missionaries through faith-infused diet and exercise. Physically, love can promote a better sex life for spouses and more vitalized fellowship for friends. When we create synergy between spiritual things such as fasting and prayer with physical things such as running and lifting, we paint a picture for all to behold in honor of Jesus Christ's name, for a greater glory to God.

> *Therefore be imitators of God, as beloved children. And walk in love, as Christ loved us and gave himself up for us, a fragrant offering and sacrifice to God.*
>
> —Eph. 5:1–2

Jesus said:

> *By this all people will know that you are my disciples, if you have love for one another.*
>
> —John 13:35

The love He spoke of was God's sacrificial love, the same love that enabled Him to lay down His life for us. When we possess that kind of love for the body God gave us and the body Jesus gave for us, we can show the world His definition of health and fitness. It should be out of God's love for our bodies that we commit to a rigorous workout routine. And it should be out of Jesus's love for our bodies that we surrender junk food and replace it with a well-balanced diet.

When the church further rises up to apply love correctly and biblically, we will indeed build a stronger body of Christ.

Faith-infused fitness will only serve to consistently replenish and increase that strength. It will produce better soldiers in the army of God, rugged warriors in the fight for faith, and steadier bearers of the cross. But without love, it will mean nothing.

CHAPTER 5

Be above Reproach

The truth hurts. Most of the time, we don't want to hear it, especially when it concerns what we eat. In a perfect world, we'd be able to eat as much as we want, drink whatever we want, and never have to worry about the consequences of our unhealthy actions. The fact is that we can't, and it's physically obvious. Today, obesity and heart disease are responsible for hundreds of billions of dollars of healthcare costs in the United States alone. More and more people are gorging themselves into high blood pressure, cancer, heart attacks, and strokes. Hundreds of thousands of deaths each year in the United States are attributed to individuals who are excessively overweight.

We Are Hurting Our Bodies

The fast-food culture has swept through the nation, from coast to coast, serving up saturated fat, high fructose corn syrup, and genetically modified organisms. Our citizens have fallen in lust with processed meats, fried potatoes, sugary sweets, and over-sized soda pop. Their attention is being drawn to advertisements promising finger-licking goodness and fresh eats through an invitation to dine in or drive through. It seems that it's all meant to make us feel alive by thinking outside the bun and having it our way with special orders for cheap. It's almost as if these quick-serve restaurants' slogans want to convince us that we deserve fast food because we've earned it.

The only thing we'll earn from living off of the super-sized combo meals and dollar menus is a free ride to the nearest emergency room. Treatment at a hospital for coronary heart disease can cost tens of thousands of dollars. So what good is it to save all that time and money mooching off the value menu? Once we end up on bed restriction, our prognosis will keep us there for days while the medical bills end up depleting our bank account.

I'd never want to put myself or my loved ones through something scary like that. If it ended up causing sudden death or loss, I know my family couldn't handle that. I have found that microwaved bacon, imitation guacamole, and fake sour cream squirted out of dispensing guns is really not worth the risk. And it's hard for me to believe that we are too busy to make home-cooked meals for our loved ones. Quality family time seems to be such a low priority these days that we just plop self-serve pizzas and Chinese take-out on the kitchen counter while everyone goes about their business, eating in separate rooms. That is the reality for too many of us neglectful parents who now have potbellied pre-teens and pudgy adolescents.

I've also found that most of our issues that relate to obesity can be self-diagnosed and prevented. I didn't need a doctor to figure out why my shirts and pants wouldn't fit anymore or why I had chest pains all the time. I just looked at what I ate and how much I exercised. I also asked my friends and fitness buddies, because I knew if they really cared about me, they'd tell me. It was awkward and uncomfortable, but I figured why not give the truth a swallow?

Plenty of Opportunity to Get Healthy

Here's some truth for you: The average person lives less than four miles from a gym. It takes just a few minutes, sometimes seconds, for us to get there. Along with the fast-food culture dominating every corner and shopping center, there has been a large wave of physical fitness centers moving into urban and suburban areas in every state. The opportunity to get fit on our own and improve our health has never been bigger.

Group fitness activities such as boot camps, aerobics, and cycling are all out there and available to us. You might have to buy a membership somewhere, but a lot of places cost as little as 10 dollars a month. Some gyms are even free. The more popular corporate chains can typically start you off with a one-week trial period before requiring you to buy a membership.

Health and wellness has become a billion-dollar industry and is quite lucrative for the private sector. Commercial gyms will rake in millions of dollars of annual revenue with a guaranteed annual increase in profit the longer they stay in business. Personal trainers can expect to close the gap between their average income and a six-figure salary. They will bank on the hype of New Year's resolutionists, marathoners, mud runners, and healthcare plans that include memberships to gyms.

Companies and organizations in all industries have also taken matters into their own hands. Those undergoing new construction or expansion are drawing up plans to include employee fitness facilities that can be utilized after hours and on lunch breaks. Others have set up reimbursement programs and allowances so their staff can offset the cost of getting in shape. Even churches are building weight rooms, basketball courts, and cardio areas adjacent to their sanctuaries in hopes of keeping their congregations vibrant.

If that doesn't work, you still have a plethora of information online. Social media is rampant with reputable workout videos, expert dietary instruction, and accredited exercise regimens from reliable sources. There are also products you can buy to use in the comfort of your own home—treadmills, exercise equipment, operative training DVDs, and downloadable fitness apps for your personal electronic devices. All these have proved to be effective and beneficial for people on a global scale.

Do We Even Want to Be Healthy?

We literally have fitness at our fingertips. Yet, every year our nation grows wider with more overweight and out-of-shape Americans, so much so that there is now a plus-size movement spreading across the United States advocating for fat acceptance. A national agenda to affirm obesity has convinced many that this alternative is a moral obligation. I agree that all people should be accepted for who they are, but not at the expense of their hearts and souls.

It seems like a lot of overweight people feel oppressed, excluded, and judged when confronted by others trying to help them with their issue. Gyms and fitness centers filled with macho men and women are too overwhelming for heavyset guys and gals. They get strange looks from those who label them as abnormally intolerable. And evidently, some fashion designers and sports apparel companies shut out most, if not all, double-extra-large folks. The health industry's attempt to care for these individuals seems to be backfiring.

As a chubby kid growing up and as someone who struggles to shed fat and put on muscle, I can relate to that feeling of isolation and rejection. I have seen how certain inner circles and private cliques discourage novices from trying to exercise in their territories. Some physically fit people only want to be around other physically fit people of similar knowledge and equivalent strength. It does seem like gyms and fitness centers are meant to attract and cater to the more athletic and already slender.

As a personal trainer, I confess it is more enjoyable to have clients who are either already in shape or don't have too much weight to lose. The beginners usually complain and often quit. Sometimes trainers don't have the patience to deal with such negativity. But we can't let the shallowness of others dictate how we feel about our bodies. The flaw in our source for motivation is that it begins with everything except God.

God Is Reason Enough for a Healthy Life

So what is our source of motivation? Is it acceptance, longevity, self-image, or self-love? Whatever it is, if it's not God, it will never be enough. Without God, there will always be a missing element to the success of our fitness, one that, when discovered, will intensify all our health and wellness efforts to the maximum. It begins with the example of a sinless savior in service to a holy God. Our bodies were made for Him, purchased by the blood of Jesus, and now the dwelling place of His Holy Spirit.

> *Or do you not know that your body is a temple of the Holy Spirit within you, whom you have from God? You are not your own, for you were bought with a price. So glorify God in your body.*
>
> —1 Cor. 6:19–20

Seeking momentum and resolve in anything less than Him as our incentive will only leave us cast out, sold short, and probably worse off than when we started. There is a higher standard that God calls holiness that we all must strive for and live by. *Holiness* is defined as staying clean and remaining disconnected from every dirty deed and shameful act, every polluted or disgusting thought, and all profanity and demeaning words in our vocabulary.

Since we have these promises, beloved, let us cleanse ourselves from every defilement of body and spirit, bringing holiness to completion in the fear of God.

—2 Cor. 7:1

When we keep our bodies free from gluttonous overeating and clean from drug addiction and alcoholism, we participate physically in the divine restoration and rejuvenation of God's people. But holiness does not make us better than anybody else, nor does it place us on a superior level. It simply reflects our genuine belief in a perfect God and confirms our desire to be sanctified by the Holy Spirit, not corrupted by the evil in the world. Making such sacrifices is evidence that we trust in God's promises and that we're truly seeking to become more like Him.

Holiness Builds Strength

Holiness is more than a religious construct; it is a condition of the body. Because God is holy, walking in His ways produces in us rock-solid confidence. That confidence in Christ can conquer any fears that may be hindering us. By conquering our fears, the Holy Spirit enters our minds and our bodies to overcome weakness. When Jesus was alive, He trained His disciples to be holy both spiritually and physically. This charge has been passed down to all those who follow Him.

You therefore must be perfect, as your heavenly Father is perfect.

—Matt. 5:48

Answering the call to holiness enables us to resist unhealthy temptations in all circumstances. Through proper diet, holiness helps us not eat what we shouldn't eat and helps us drink in moderation as we should. It's quite common in our communities to visit restaurants packed with remiss overeaters and bars filled with heavy drinkers. Our demeanor will either show approval of such behavior or reveal a setting apart that resembles God as our source of motivation in everything.

> *Therefore, preparing your minds for action, and being sober-minded, set your hope fully on the grace that will be brought to you at the revelation of Jesus Christ. As obedient children, do not be conformed to the passions of your former ignorance, but as he who called you is holy, you also be holy in all your conduct.*
>
> —1 Pet. 1:13–15

This concept emanates from the infallible attributes of God, who derives glory from His creation. So we must do all we can to glorify Him with our bodies. Jesus had zero sinful cravings and was never gluttonous, only blameless. So, too, must we conduct ourselves in a way that others find zero fault. Since the Holy Spirit is never idle or lazy but always providing strength and empowerment, so, too, we must also stay active, pursuing strength and our utmost for His highest. Too many of us are unfamiliar with this idea of God's holiness building our strength. The real issue is our heart. Even with a gym and a fitness center on every corner or mass production of in-home exercise equipment, the actual issue still needs to be addressed. How many gym memberships do you think get cancelled after 30 days or go unused for years at a time?

How many weights and barbells end up in storage? How many treadmills and ab machines end up in a garage sale? Too many to count.

The real issue is hardly ever talked about because it calls into question our lifestyle and our preferred way of thinking. We will never overcome what we won't confront, and what we refuse to confront is our dependence on God for everything.

Our Priorities Are Out of Whack

Before I considered my calling and purpose in life, I never thought of submitting my will to God or abstaining from anything for His sake. I focused more on sowing and reaping for my own elation and benefit. That was why my refrigerator was stocked with beer, butter, and biscuits. My freezer was stuffed with ice cream and hamburger patties, my pantry with potato chips and powdered donuts. I wanted big screen TVs throughout the whole house, closets full of high-dollar clothes and shoes I'd never wear. A simple mode of transportation wasn't going to cut it. I had to have a sports car *and* a truck, a motorbike *and* a boat.

I wanted to be the master of all things, not a lowly servant. I wanted to be a self-assertive king, not a mere shepherd. I spent more and gave less, working hard for purchasing power and financial security as my safeguard. What I didn't realize was that quite often, material things provided me with a false sense of well-being, pushing me further away from God. Then I dismissed holiness altogether, as if God were unnecessary and expendable.

Naturally, we want to be lords over our own lives. Even those of us who have obtained saving faith can struggle with being impartial to God. How often do we think about being above reproach? I know I never used to. I just wanted to fit into the norm and be well-thought-of by others according to my good deeds. It's hard for some of us to pay attention to our health and fitness when we have so much other stuff going on.

It seems like our most pressing priorities are work, bills, rent, television shows, social media, and just hangin' out. If we get around to exercise or physical activity, it's typically one or two days a week. I call that "feeding the gym my leftovers." I used to just jog on a treadmill in front of a mounted television screen. Or I'd plug my ears with hyped up music to distract myself from how out of breath I was and how painful it was to just be there.

I would sweat all over the StairMaster thinking, *My God, when will this be over?* I'd fantasize about what my next meal would be. I'd think about how much I deserved a large soda and a bacon double cheeseburger, a bottle of wine with lasagna, or a margarita with nachos. The struggle is real, and we all go through it.

But in those difficulties, we aren't turning to God for strength. We're turning to the idea of rewarding ourselves with euphoric highs no matter what the cost or consequence. That idea dates back to the start of the human race—with Adam and Eve. When the devil convinced Eve to eat the forbidden fruit, she mistakenly perceived that it would be more satisfying than obedience to God.

Our Bodies Crave Junk

We cannot study the original sin passage in Genesis chapter 3 enough. It reveals so much about who we are—terribly deep down in our core. The Bible says the fall of humankind was the result of Adam and Eve's touching, tasting, and eating what God had strictly prohibited. Stunningly, every sin is related and connected to a desired fulfillment for the body. Whether it's the pleasure of tacos for a full stomach, the numbing effect of tequila for stress, or the joy of being high on illegal substances—all of them are either inhaled, consumed, or devoured for sensual purposes.

But the call to be holy and above reproach goes way beyond what we put in our bodies.

> *Hear me, all of you, and understand: There is nothing outside a person that by going into him can defile him, but the things that come out of a person are what defile him.*
>
> —Mark 7:14–15

Jesus taught that it is not what goes into the body that makes a person gross, nasty, or despicable, but rather what comes out of the body through the heart. More than the precautionary measures in choosing what we eat or drink is the attitude behind why we eat or drink. So, we ought to be inwardly concerned about self-control and outwardly focused on the example we set as followers of Christ. What are we thinking about when we stuff our faces with junk food or drink or smoke too much? Keeping physical obedience to God in the forefront of our minds is essential for staying in step with the Holy Spirit to break unhealthy habits.

A big part of being fit is living by the godly standard of internal cleanliness so the power and glory of Christ can shine externally to those around us. If we're going to be fit, we must begin with an internal approach rather than an external approach. We needn't be concerned with how to lose weight until we've discovered why we put it on in the first place.

Was it because of stress, carelessness, laziness, or all of the above? We shouldn't want to add muscle to our bodies until we've had the chance to consider exactly why we think we need it. Is it for vain purposes or selfish gain? Do we have theological reasons stemming from a godly mindset to desire stronger, healthier bodies?

The Definition of Fitness

Contrary to popular belief, fitness is not defined as bulging biceps and six-pack abs. Strength, power, energy, and endurance are all perfectly demonstrated by God who has no body. Fitness is defined by the cultivation of God's grace, the transfer of Jesus's strength, and the refinement of the Holy Spirit's empowerment in us and through us. Scripture spells this out in no uncertain terms.

But he said to me, "My grace is sufficient for you, for my power is made perfect in weakness." Therefore I will boast all the more gladly of my weaknesses, so that the power of Christ may rest upon me. For the sake of Christ, then, I am content with weaknesses . . . hardships. . . . For when I am weak, then I am strong.

—2 Cor. 12:9–10

We can attain perfect bodies on the outside, but without abiding love, sustaining self-control, and a longing for holiness, we will never be as fit as the overweight people who are on their knees, pleading to God for help with diet and exercise. We might have the fastest metabolism and the greatest athleticism, but if our pursuit of fitness is self-centered and not Christ-centered, we will never be as healthy as the hefty men and women who present their bodies as living sacrifices in worship. Health always includes holiness.

But what if we have already submitted to Christ and are denying ourselves daily? Why, then, are we still tipping the scales toward obesity? Each of us wakes up in the morning and prays to God for a good day. We ought to add a prayer for Him to empower us to make healthy choices as well. We implore Him for protection from harm, lust, and the devil, for example. We should also pray to God for protection from overeating and excessive junk food cravings.

We pray to God sincerely for strength at work to meet deadlines, complete projects, and cope with our bosses. God can also give us that same strength to work out and exercise. We pray to Him for endurance in the balance between work life, social life, and family life. God can also give us endurance to add gym life to that balance. Prayer gives us direct access to God through Jesus Christ. He has made a commitment to us to provide all that we need. Within the call to holiness, if we ask in His name for stronger bodies to be healthier vessels, He will make it happen for us.

Whatever you ask in my name, this I will do, that the Father may be glorified in the Son. If you ask me anything in my name, I will do it.

—John 14:13–14

We Must Hold Each Other Accountable

A big part of answering the call to be above reproach is, again, depending on God for everything. But we must also be humble enough to ask for everything—not to just help us with things such as making more money and having more success, but also to help us care for our bodies since the body is God's temple. Being a Christ-like example to others with our bodies encourages them to do the same and is one way we can responsibly cultivate camaraderie.

Keeping each other accountable can be difficult when no one wants to be put on the spot, especially when it comes to their physical appearance and shape. But if someone we care about, friend or family member, suddenly packs on 20 pounds of unhealthy fat, we should draw them out—in love—with tough questions about how and why. Remember, we can't overcome what we won't confront. If we care for one another as we care for ourselves, we can trust in God for an outcome that will lessen the awkwardness, bring strengthening, and diminish the offense that takes place as we lovingly call each other out.

Accountability is most effective when we can achieve it spiritually and physically. There has to be complete transparency among the people of God as we strive for holiness together. Think of it this way. We all have friends, relatives, loved ones, people we care about who can sometimes act like jerks or be mean or rude. Some of them can be cruel and crude, complainers, and nasty gossips. Yet we'll tolerate their slander, their foul mouths, and impoliteness until it becomes unbearable.

Eventually, we reach a breaking point and address the issue. We ask them why they're so mean or why they always have bad things to say about people. Sometimes, we have to be blunt and confrontational. Some of us even bring witnesses or get help from others to back us up. We'll schedule an intervention or counseling or a meeting with someone they trust for correction. The point is that it is our custom to deal with each other's emotional shortcomings.

It's easy to appeal to each other about our emotional shortcomings, especially when it affects us. In love, we say things like, "That was rude, and you should apologize," or "Hey, your attitude is wrong, so let's work together to fix it." Most of us have genuine concern in these moments because we want to keep the peace. The idea of righting wrongs and saying sorry comes from the biblical principle of forgiveness and repentance. It's how we conduct ourselves when we deal with conflict resolution. We understand that it is our responsibility to look out for one another in those instances and build each other up by caring about people's feelings, but most importantly, to protect them from wrongdoing.

The same biblical logic applies to our physical shortcomings that affect all of us directly. We are all one body, the body of Christ. If we're not functioning properly as the body of Christ, ministry cannot reach its full potential. Only with strong legs can we walk the extra mile with the same compassion as the good Samaritan. Only with strong bodies can we wholeheartedly show the light and love of Christ to the lost. As easy as it is to help those struggling with profanity, anger, anxiety, and depression, we should be just as loving and caring to help each other in times of gluttony, idleness, laziness, and all other unhealthy behaviors.

Leaders Set the Example for Health and Fitness

When it comes to physical appearance, nobody wants to be critiqued, so we don't even go there. I can remember being embarrassed about my body. It was hard for me to point out other people's weight problems when I had a huge spare tire around my waist. They would just point the finger back at me. That is part of the issue. Being overweight is too common an occurrence and too touchy a subject, so we carry on, tolerating each other's unhealthy weight gain. But, this is one area of our lives that urgently needs reform, and it starts at the top.

In the church, spiritual change begins with leadership—and so should physical change. Overseers, pastors, and elders whose qualifications include self-control should definitely be prepared to model good eating habits if they are going to provide biblical counsel for gluttony. Leaders in the congregation who serve as examples and have the most influence should definitely make an effort to stay in shape. Within the call to be blameless is a responsibility to outwardly demonstrate that we are free from addiction, obsessive craving, and laziness. If we are going to profess that our bodies are the temples of God's Holy Spirit, then we should be diligent to be as protective of our bodies as we are of our souls and the souls of others.

> *For if your brother is grieved by what you eat, you are no longer walking in love. By what you eat, do not destroy the one for whom Christ died. Do not, for the sake of food, destroy the work of God. Everything is indeed clean, but it is wrong for anyone to make another stumble by what he eats.*
> —Rom. 14:15, 20

Fitness movements such as the non-religious types of yoga and secular groups of CrossFit will become increasingly attractive to churchgoers if pastors don't model good health and fitness. Leaders must all be aware of what the Bible says about food, healthy living, diet, and nutrition. When church leaders are able to speak into their brothers' and sisters' lives about these things, they build stronger trust within the church and magnify Christ who sets the example for us in all things.

Right now, there are secular fitness groups of highly self-motivated individuals making members of every denomination feel energized and refreshed. I used to be in one of them. Instead of considering the possibility of exercising in a community with believers, I signed up for communal bonding in a sweatbox full of complete strangers. I was sharing worldly physical goals by detaching my faith from fitness, and it worked for me temporarily. But as a result, I was saying yes to myself rather than yes to a holy God.

I'm not suggesting that Christians close themselves off from the outside world of fitness. But if the invitation to worldly transformation can produce change, how much more should Christ's call to godly transformation bring about change. If mud runs and Spartan races can inspire people and achieve results with temporal things, how much more will holiness transform and inspire with eternal things. The power of self-love, self-belief, and self-confidence will never be as strong as faith in Jesus, love for God, and the power of the Holy Spirit!

The Church's Strength Is at Stake

Put off your old self, which belongs to your former manner of life and is corrupt through deceitful desires, and . . . be renewed in the spirit of your minds, and . . . put on the new self, created after the likeness of God in true righteousness and holiness.

—Eph. 4:22–24

Putting off the old self is one of my favorite biblical principles. It's how we build a stronger church, and we need to be a stronger church. We need strong leaders to make strong disciples of all nations, people who can tirelessly help the homeless and less fortunate, care for widows and orphans with vibrance, and better serve our communities without growing weary.

> *Seek the LORD and his strength; seek his presence continually!*
> —1 Chron. 16:11

The call to be above reproach is a call to a sacrifice of time and energy. The power of God is at our disposal to put an end to the death and destruction caused by heart attacks, strokes, cancers, diseases, and other physically crippling disorders. Every one of us, church leader or not, has a responsibility to answer the call to holiness by caring for our bodies and caring for the bodies of the church. We are all together the body of Christ, one big family. Let's be a strong, healthy family. Let's start living it out together. Let's minimize the catnaps and chill sessions to spend more time meeting the physical needs of others. Instead of raising our families on fast food and sit-down restaurants, let's set aside time to shop for whole foods and cook healthier options. I'm done starving myself with juice fasts and crash diets to slim down. I want God's holiness to help me plan my meals with consistency and make time for rigorous exercise. When our physical traits collectively resemble Spirit-filled lives and our physical duties harmoniously resemble service to Christ, we honor each other, and we honor our God. We provide an environment that beckons saintship into our lives and reveals the marks of true Christianity to the lives of the lost. The truth doesn't have to hurt, and being above reproach doesn't have to be a pain. There's no reason to be scared of set-apartness because we're not living for ourselves. We're living for our maker daily and hourly. And in the energized charge toward holiness, every second counts.

CHAPTER 6

Master Plan for Your Body

Have you ever designed or invented anything? Is there something grand in your life that you personally put together piece by piece, brick by brick, like a house or an intricate machine? The process can be a bit time-consuming. Along with tons of effort, new construction and smart engineering demand energy, diligence, patience, meticulous planning, and calculation.

Building something requires knowledge, passion, and a well-thought-out strategy or blueprint. The process requires a step-by-step order to completion with the primary parts that need to be assembled in place before you achieve the finished product. Then once it's accomplished, you take a step back, and just by looking at it, it's crystal-clear that someone made it and forged it to serve a purpose.

God's Design Has Been Taken for Granted

Wherever you are right now, take a look around. What do you see? Tables and chairs, sidewalks and buildings, planes, trains, automobiles—all these were made with a purpose. Coffee cups and laptops, refrigerators and microwaves—they were all designed with intent to do something for us.

But these things are so common that we don't even think about the behind-the-scenes labor that went into their mass production. We don't even want to know how they work. All we care about is that they're functional and provide something useful and convenient. We take them for granted while it seems there is an endless supply. If one malfunctions, breaks down, or is lost or stolen, we simply replace it with another one.

Tragically, the same can be said about us—people in general. We have forgotten our inventor, our designer, and have therefore forgotten that everyone on this planet serves a specific purpose, including us. Take another look around. Whom do you see? Somebody's father or mother? Someone's son or daughter? I wasn't always aware that God designs, determines, and develops us to fulfill a destiny. I never saw how complete strangers could do anything for me. I just viewed them as insignificant human beings. I didn't really care who they were unless they could provide me with some benefit or accommodation.

Until they provided some degree of service, extended courtesy, or satisfaction to prove their significance in making my life better, they were just people taking up air and space. So why tolerate them? Why put up with another person making the grocery store line slower and longer, another idiot driver clogging up the freeway with traffic, another incompetent cashier at the drive-through window, and yet another homeless bum by the stop sign? These people are worthless, right? Wrong!

Satan Hates God's Design for Our Bodies

Such was the arrogant condition and narcissistic personality disorder of Satan. He held my body captive until God set me free from his bondage. Some call him the devil, the enemy, the tempter, the fallen angel. He is real, and he's out to make everyone a slave to sin, a servant of his purpose. Scripture describes Satan as one of the best looking, highest-ranking angels in all of heaven. But it wasn't enough for him. He desired more power and exaltation, even higher than God. That's when God legitimately kicked him out heaven and removed him from his position. Satan was condemned to hell for all eternity, which is the due penalty for attempting to overthrow God.

In Satan's vengeful madness, he decided to start a rebellion by influencing others to do the same, bringing forth misery and death to earth, which was a peaceful created order. He refused to acknowledge God as sovereign ruler. All he cared about was his own selfish plot to sabotage the throne of God. Right now, he and his army of demons continue to wreak havoc in all parts of the world through senseless violence, terrorism, and hate. The devil thrives on heinous acts committed everywhere, delighting in the fact that we now worship other gods and turn to other forms of joy and pleasure than what is found only in our creator.

He was a murderer from the beginning, and does not stand in truth, because there is no truth in him. When he lies, he speaks out of his own character, for he is a liar and the father of lies.

—John 8:44

His first victim was Eve, the first woman on earth. Here we are, back in Genesis Chapter 3, the fall of humankind, the incident where Satan became the concocter of all deceit. That is where God's master plan for our good was corrupted by the devil's plan for evil. With Eve as his first target, the devil tricked her into using her body for something that was never supposed to be: disobedience. When he deceived Eve, she not only committed a spiritual disobedience, causing violence to her soul, but also a physical disobedience that resulted in the breakdown of her well-being as well as ours.

So when the woman saw that the tree was good for food, and that it was a delight to the eyes, and that the tree was to be desired to make one wise, she took of its fruit and ate.

—Gen. 3:6

Not only did she think that what Satan told her was true, but she confirmed it by using her hands to grab it and her mouth to eat it.

Many in the world are still believing the devil's lies. We have been blinded by a slippery snake, a wolf out to devour sheep. He can certainly pull the wool over our eyes but never over the eyes of our shepherd. Every day, God is saving souls because He sent His son into the world with a specific purpose, and he is setting us free from the devil's captivity. His mission was foretold to be a spiritual restorer of our souls and simultaneously a physical restorer of our bodies.

Strengthen the weak hands, and make firm the feeble knees. Say to those who have an anxious heart, "Be strong; fear not! Behold, your God will come with vengeance, with the recompense of God. He will come and save you." Then the eyes of the blind shall be opened, and the ears of the deaf unstopped; then shall the lame man leap like a deer, and the tongue of the mute sing for joy.

—Isa. 35:3–6

Jesus Restores Our Body's Design

Such was the vision, the heart, and the passion of Jesus Christ. My body and soul are now His; my name is engraved on His hands. Some people call Him lord, savior, son of God, or Messiah. He is real, and He's out to make everyone a soldier set free from sin, a servant of His purpose. Jesus was God in the flesh, but He never took advantage of His power and authority.

Instead, He humbled Himself. He led by example in godliness beyond compare as a servant to others, in full obedience to God, even when He knew it would cost Him His life. God sent Jesus into this world to die for us. He died for our lack of self-control to remedy our gluttony, our laziness, our sinful cravings, and our addictions. And He did so willingly. By His spirit, He transmits His holiness to us, making our bodies His vessels.

We have been empowered to use our whole physical being to imitate His life and what He stood for, in word and deed, through duty and service. By taking care of our bodies, we participate in the supernatural activity of God's full restoration, catalyzing testimonial evidences of grace in our lives. So instead of touching what is forbidden, like the mistake Adam and Eve made, we use our hands to do the ministry of Christ. Instead of using our mouths to taste what God has prohibited, like the mistake Adam and Eve made, we eat only what our God has deemed permissible.

Eat According to God's Design

To do that, we must examine food according to its lawfulness and its helpfulness. Taking fruit from the tree of the knowledge of good and evil wasn't lawful for Eve to do. Neither was it helpful to Adam or anyone else born after the fall. Our bodies were made to perfectly reflect God's image, so we can't just go around eating whatever we feel like eating. The day Eve decided to eat what was unlawful, her health began to deteriorate. The moment Adam ate what was unhelpful, his fitness was subject to decline.

God provides us with a world filled with wonderful food and the means to prepare delicious dishes. But we must partake of our food with the attitude that every decision we make with our bodies further unites us to Him. It also should increasingly unite us to each other so we can grow in strength, love, and harmony together. God's word speaks to us about the healthiest way to do that.

> *"All things are lawful," but not all things are helpful. "All things are lawful," but not all things build up. Let no one seek his own good, but the good of his neighbor. Eat whatever is sold in the meat market without raising any question on the ground of conscience. For "the earth is the Lord's and the fullness thereof."*
>
> —1 Cor. 10:23–26

How do we decide what is lawful? Everything is lawful, except cannibalism. Chicken, pork, beef, fish, shrimp, turkey, duck, and lamb are some common main course items that God created for us, just to name a few. If you can eat them in faith with a clear conscience, that's great. Just be mindful of portion size, nutrition facts, and how you season or prepare your meals. Chicken fried steak, for example, is always going to be worse for you than a grilled steak. Likewise, baked potatoes will always be a healthier option than French fries.

Be cautious of artificial flavors, additives, and genetically modified foods. Never forget that God's creation was designed to be organic and whole, and we are meant to be of sound mind and body.

You really can't go wrong with fruits, vegetables, and nuts, but pay attention to sugar intake, caloric intake, how often you snack, and the reasons why you snack. As you put your meals together with balance, think quality, not quantity. Remember to listen to the Holy Spirit and your body so you don't eat past the point of satiation. There isn't anything wrong with not clearing your plate or with skipping dessert.

As a young boy, my siblings and I were taught to finish all our food. What I teach my children is somewhat similar to a technique found in the Okinawan diet, Hara Hachi Bu, which is simply to stop eating when you're 80 percent full. This is one technique we use to prevent the constant stretching of our stomachs and avoid putting on excess weight. It also is a practical way to help us remember that our bodies belong to God and remind us to pay close attention to what the scripture says.

Gracious words are like a honeycomb, sweetness to the soul and health to the body.

—Prov.16:24

With the Holy Spirit as our guide, we allow Him to educate us on what's helpful in the physical sense by examining the effect foods have on our bodies and the bodies of the people we eat with. But also, we pay close attention to how our minds and their minds are affected in the spiritual sense. Eating beef or lamb all the time might make you fat and lazy, but it might make others strong and energetic. Eating fish might keep you lean and happy, but it could also make others cranky or moody. We need to be discerning about these things as we pray for direction in our own diets and in the eating habits of our friends and family.

Most of what I used to eat came in a sealed box or bag. I never prayerfully considered how much of it I should consume or the amount I would feed to others. As a Christian, I believe we have to be concerned with what we eat but not as much as how we eat it. Double-cheeseburgers, burritos, and pizza used to be my sustenance, and my kids lived off Lunchables and Happy Meals. What I saw in my life was a lack of stewardship for my body and theirs by never considering healthier alternatives. Once I learned that God has a plan for all our bodies, I became more aware of the compromising convenience of processed foods.

We were not designed to be greedy little pigs. We are like sheep living in a healthy environment under the care and nourishment of our shepherd, Jesus.

> *For thus says the LORD God: Behold, I, I myself will search for my sheep and will seek them out. . . . I will feed them with good pasture, and on the mountain heights of Israel shall be their grazing land. . . . I will seek the lost, and I will bring back the strayed, and I will bind up the injured, and I will strengthen the weak, and the fat and the strong I will destroy. I will feed them in justice. . . . Is it not enough for you to feed on the good pasture? . . . I myself will judge between the fat sheep and the lean sheep.*
>
> —Ezek. 34:11, 14, 16, 18, 20

As God watches over us, His desire is for us to be spiritually restored to Him and to be physically restored for Him. Our purpose includes spiritually feeding others while being spiritually fed with wisdom and physically feeding others while being physically fed in wisdom. God wants us to be a people of hospitality and generosity. When we feed on the good pasture, fighting over restaurant tables ceases, the shoving and trampling at grocery stores diminishes, and those who are starving get attention from those of us who have way too much to eat.

Enjoy Freedom the Healthy Way

Are we free in Christ to eat and drink whatever we want? Absolutely! God loves it when our thirst and hunger are satisfied to His glory, but not at the neglect of our spiritual and physical well-being. The problem occurs when we take it overboard and subject various parts of our bodies to imbalances, such as chemically in the brain.

There is nothing spiritually or physically good about postprandial somnolence—commonly known as "food coma." Food comas decrease conscious awareness and activate lethargy while throwing off the way your body uses protein and energy. Blood flow to the brain is diverted and makes you tired and sleepy. Imagine doing this to yourself three times a day, and then you can easily see how it presents a problem to health and fitness.

Jesus has declared all foods clean, and Paul the apostle wisely instructs us that we must never put lawful things into our bodies at an indulgent rate. Careless eating and binge drinking cause damage to our bodies and can turn us into alcoholics and food addicts if we're not careful. We must be cautious to digest nothing that would take God's place as the highest and ultimate satisfier.

> *"All things are lawful for me," but not all things are helpful. "All things are lawful for me," but I will not be dominated by anything.*
> —1 Cor. 6:12

Since God is our source of true fulfillment, wisdom says to seek His ways in what we eat for breakfast, lunch, and dinner. Since God is our source of true contentment, seeking His counsel regarding our workouts and exercise programs honors Him as creator. Utilizing our bodies in devotion to His will and purpose with enthusiasm and energy is an indelible mark of a true Christ follower.

God has created and purposed us to imitate Him, to chase after His attributes and character. Aligning our minds, souls, and bodies to resemble Jesus is a beautiful display of our faith and our desire to be like Him. This alignment demonstrates the strong connection and unbreakable bond that exists within those who love Him. It's like children aspiring to be like their parents and make them proud, embracing the inheritance of their family name. When we as brothers and sisters in Christ make good choices regarding the strength of our minds and the health of our bodies, we testify of His goodness as father and His greatness as lord.

After God's Own Heart

There was once a man named David who reigned as king over all Israel. You probably know him best from the story of David and Goliath in which he struck down the nation of Israel's most fearsome enemy with a slingshot and a single stone. It was a battle that spawned a wave of prosperity for David and would be remembered for all time. During his fight with Goliath, there was a short dialogue just before he prevailed over the Philistine champion. David said:

> *"This day the LORD will deliver you into my hand, and I will strike you down . . . and that all this assembly may know that the LORD saves."*
> —1 Sam. 17:46–47

From that day forward, David was known as a warrior, heroic leader, and courageous man of faith. But his most unique quality is that he is remembered as a man after God's own heart. No other king throughout biblical history was ever described as a man after God's own heart or thought of in that way.

What made David so special? Surely, he had his share of shortcomings, spiritually and physically. He definitely struggled. But he was also a longsuffering, merciful, and forgiving man. He was a king who loved his enemies when they didn't deserve it.

Distinct from all other monarchs, he quickly admitted his faults. Unlike Adam, who blamed Eve for his sin, David experienced great blessing and hallowing since he was consistent in taking responsibility for his actions and confessing his wrongdoings to God. David also showed compassion to many and forgave many. He was filled with an endless desire to know God, praise God, and worship Him. As a man after God's own heart, he yearned for the spiritual and physical restoration that only his lord and savior could provide.

In Psalm 144, David sings praise about God's master plan for our bodies and His created order. God is our foundation for everything in life, and it is God who prepares us physically for the work He has for us to do. He is always our source of strength and protection from the unlawful and the unhelpful. David was aware of all this. He also knew that it was God who made him king and gave him his authority on earth.

> *Blessed be the* LORD, **my rock, who trains my hands for war, and my fingers for battle**; *he is my steadfast love and* **my fortress, my stronghold and my deliverer, my shield** *and he in whom I take refuge, who subdues peoples under me.*
>
> —Ps. 144:1–2

God is a divine warrior who fought for righteousness in the case of David and his enemies. In my case, God helped me fight against the enemy within. Whenever I was tempted to drown myself in alcoholism or binge eat due to stress and depression, the Holy Spirit was there to keep me on course. As Satan deceived Eve to eat what was forbidden, the nonbelieving world led me astray with seemingly harmless fun and shameless debauchery. For the longest time, I was convinced that lying, cheating, and stealing were okay, denying that my mind, hands, and mouth were made for integrity, truth, and fruitfulness.

> *Stretch out your hand from on high; rescue me and deliver me from the many waters, from the hand of foreigners, whose mouths speak lies and whose right hand is a right hand of falsehood.*
>
> —Ps. 144:7–8

We Were Designed for Good Health

Although an imperfect man, David put all his trust in God, which was why he got down on his knees to pray and worship God in times of need. David would often plead with God to help him in his weakness, giving thanks and praise to Him as he received God's blessing and deliverance.

> *I will sing a new song to you, O God; upon a ten-stringed harp I will play to you, who gives victory to kings, who rescues David his servant from the cruel sword.*
>
> —Ps. 144:9–10

David was fully aware that his soul belonged to his maker and that he was bodily God's design, set apart for a monumental purpose. He loved God and God's Holy Spirit. Humbled by his own sinful nature, David knew that nothing he received from God was ever deserved but that God had found favor with him because of his heart. He knew God was perfect in every way and therefore sought to make Him known as the perfect creator.

David possessed a desire to free the world from enslavement by proclaiming and restoring the name of God, who originally created us for good and for the good of others. He made us to walk the earth in perfect bliss, to be flawlessly strong and faultlessly competent, enjoying our families in good health with bountiful food and plentiful pleasure. That was David's vision throughout this fabulous psalm of great renown.

> *May our sons in their youth be like plants full grown, our daughters like corner pillars cut for the structure of a palace; may our granaries be full, providing all kinds of produce; may our sheep bring forth thousands and ten thousands in our fields; may our cattle be heavy with young,*

suffering no mishap or failure in bearing; may there be no cry of distress in our streets! Blessed are the people to whom such blessings fall! Blessed are the people whose God is the LORD!

—Ps. 144:12–15

Jesus Loves God's Design for Our Bodies

God sent Jesus to fulfill this beautiful vision of good health and thriving humanity in Christ, orchestrating the proper time and place to carry out His mission. With specific objectives, Jesus carried out that redemptive conquest—first, by being the perfect example of the master plan for our bodies, and second, by sacrificing His unblemished body to be the perfect mediator between us and God—so we could be reconciled to Him, reborn as a new creation in Christ.

When we believe, Jesus's righteousness of both His body and His soul is transferred to us, along with the cancellation and eradication of our wrongdoings. And now, God has exalted Jesus higher than any other name in all of heaven and earth. Our bodies are spiritually and physically attached to His name through faith. The plan is to one day be glorified with Him in perfect, everlasting health.

Throughout Jesus's ministry, He declared a revolution of radical faith, influencing many to believe, performing miraculous physical healings, bringing mercy and life to an oppressed people. Jesus came to teach us that He is the way, the truth, and the life. He is the *way* because He provided the perfect body for our spiritual restoration. He is the *truth* because He is the bona fide son of the irrefutable God. He is the *life* because in Him, we are spiritually and physically restored as new creations.

Jesus made blind men see and crippled people walk. He turned immoral mistresses into women of purity and transformed religious nose-punchers into gracious peacemakers.

Jesus can do the same for you as you do this:

Train yourself for godliness.

—1 Tim. 4:7

And as you do this:

Work out your own salvation with fear and trembling, for it is God who works in you, both to will and to work for his good pleasure.

—Phil. 2:12–13

Jesus helped me embrace the new self by teaching me to humbly ask God what His original intent was for my body when He created me, but also, as a redeemed soul and His temple, to continuously listen to what God's master plan is for my body going forward. When I examined all the things I did with my body as my old self, I compared them to the actions, deeds, and fruit of the Holy Spirit. What I saw was a huge disconnect, a long history of compromise and hypocrisy.

Live with the End in View

There was a bigger picture I never thought about, a deeper meaning to life that was way beyond what I saw at surface level. I was going through life as if it were meant to be spent on a few buffets interspersed with drunken parties. I was using my hands to hoard like a squirrel, and my mouth to eat like a pig at a trough. My appetite was foolish, like a dog eating its own vomit. If my stomach and my midsection could have spoken during that time, I guarantee you they would have testified to the unlawful and unhelpful things I put into my body.

There's a better, more pleasurable way to live that brings unending joy and satisfaction. It is through God's word, as Job says:

I have treasured the words of his mouth more than my portion of food.
—Job 23:12

And it is through God's will, as Jesus says:

"My food is to do the will of him who sent me and to accomplish his work."
—John 4:34

His word and His will are what we must turn to for all things concerning our bodies, not drugs and alcohol, not pork rinds and doughnuts. Our source to carry on, to endure, to relieve stress, to quench thirst and satisfy hunger is the one who created our bodies and breathed His spirit into our nostrils, giving life to every part of us.

Our hands were designed to bring praise and honor to God, to be used for good everywhere we are, whether at work, at play, in relationships, or caring for our families. Our hands manage the ground He gave us to walk on and build and construct homes in the world He gave us. Our arms and our shoulders were made to help us do the heavy lifting, to carry crates of food for the poor, bags of clothes for the naked, and boxes of medicine for the sick. These are all things that require a congregation to have vibrance and energy. Our feet were designed for us to stand in awe of our marvelous creator and be amazed in the presence of Jesus. Let us use our mouths to confess and our voices to sing of His love for us, to shout and cheer for His victory. But we must not do this just among ourselves. Our legs were designed for community, to walk and travel to where others are, to go to those who are lost and in desperate need of His gospel, to run to every corner of the earth, leaping for joy with the urgent message that Jesus gives eternal life and everyone who calls on the name of the Lord will be saved.

That is what our bodies were created for. And God gives us our own mind to know it, our own eyes to see it, our own ears to hear it, and our own hearts to believe it. But that's not all. He gave us His son and His Holy Spirit. He has held nothing back from us so we, His people, may know that He is alive in us.

And we must be alive in Him. When we live in the image of God, we stand out from those living for their own self-image. When we can see past individuality and self-expression to live according to God's design, we can be transformed by His grace and majesty. That is how we worship Him, by offering our minds, bodies, and souls as living sacrifices to Him. Only then can the whole world take a step back and, just by looking at us, know that He has forged us to serve a purpose.

CHAPTER 7

Anatomy of Grace

Grace matters most. I can recall the first bone I ever broke in my body. I was working as a front-end loader operator at a small, family-owned rock quarry in San Diego, California. I was young and ambitious, wanting to show an exemplary work ethic by accomplishing my tasks with speed and intensity as the Marines had instilled in me. One morning, while trying to get our operation ahead of schedule, I was moving faster than normal, unknowingly sacrificing safety awareness. While pushing through a mound of crushed rock, I found some rather large debris I knew could potentially flatten a tire or cause foreign object damage to our equipment, so I jumped down off the loader to manually pick it up.

Still trying to finish my duties early in impressive fashion, I quickly climbed back into the cab of my loader and sat in the driver's seat. Without paying attention, I reached over to shut the door. But instead of grabbing the handle to close it, I grabbed the sharp metal locking mechanism that slides forward as the door slams shut. Instantly, this heavy-duty bar crushed right through my finger, cutting through the bone, yet somehow leaving my skin intact. Blood immediately spilled out as my fingernail dangled off the tip. It was gross. I screamed louder than someone being killed in a horror flick.

My supervisor hurriedly came to me as I somehow managed to get to the ground with one hand. It was obvious something was broken, so we drove straight to the emergency room. I'll never forget the ride to the hospital, for two reasons. One, there is nothing quite like the traumatizing distress of the pain of a broken bone. And two, in that moment, something spiritual happened. As a Christian man and a forgiven sinner, I began to appreciate and understand more about the physical pain that Jesus endured on the cross. In my shock and in tears, God spoke to me about what He and His son have suffered as a result of my waywardness away from my maker.

Out of Grace God Speaks

I went from conjuring up curse words in this annoying situation, asking myself *Why me?* to seeing the image of a bloody, broken savior with nails in His hands and feet and asking, *Why Him?* It was obvious that I didn't feel I deserved this baneful mishap, but before I could blame God, the Holy Spirit reminded me to trust in the master's plan for my body and life. It was sad how quickly I lost sight of this beautiful truth—that God is watching over me. How shallow my faith appeared to be in the temptation to grumble and complain.

I was ready to hold God responsible, not only for my broken finger, but for the severe inconvenience and the major setback to my upcoming plans and schedule. I knew the healing process would take months, which meant unwanted time off from work and no pay. Bills would soon pile up, and I became overwhelmed with anxiety thinking about my finances. Yet somehow, Jesus was able to calm my heart, lessen my worry, and take away my fear.

With my eyes closed tightly through the pain and the tears, I could see Jesus with His crown of thorns, carrying His heavy wooden cross to His death, determined to set me free from all my future fear and doubt. With my ears tuned in to take heed of my lord and savior, I could hear His gracious words echoing in my mind:

Father forgive them, for they know not what they do.

—Luke 23:34

I didn't think God was inflicting pain on me to teach me a lesson, but I do believe that He revealed to me what I had been seeking—a deeper understanding of what being a recipient of His mercy actually means. I lacked an amazement for His grace. Grace had become a loose term that was easy to sing about in church but so easy to take for granted the rest of the time. In that moment of pain and discomfort, the Holy Spirit spoke to me about the unsurpassed longsuffering nature of God and the incomparable pain Jesus suffered on our behalf.

God began to suffer the day we chose to disobey Him, at the fall of humankind documented and described in Genesis chapter three. So much can be said about the pain and grief we've caused God by taking a closer look at this passage and seeing the utter misuse of the human body. Digging more deeply into its tragic nature helps us see the regrettable offense to God, but it also provides answers to many of life's questions about what *really* happened at the fall and the implications of it.

God Revives through Grace

Before sin entered the world through Adam and Eve, God revealed Himself as magnificent creator and author of life. He sustains life by His power over all things through His provision of all things and in His perfect love for all things as the giver of all things. Since we were made in the image of God, we share His essential characteristics— the ability to make decisions, the power of choice, and the desire to love. But after the fall of humankind, God's character was further revealed as gracious and just. Understanding the properties of God's justice and God's grace is a big part of pursuing health and fitness. It teaches us to start back at square one with our situation at its worst.

And you were dead in the trespasses and sins in which you once walked, following the course of this world, following the prince of the power of the air, the spirit that is now at work in the sons of disobedience—among whom we all once lived in the passions of our flesh, carrying out the desires of the body and the mind, and were by nature children of wrath, like the rest of mankind. But God, being rich in mercy, because of the great love with which he loved us, even when we were dead in our trespasses, made us alive together with Christ—by grace you have been saved.

—Eph. 2:1–5

Grace is a fundamental attribute of our Christian walk. Grace empowers us to be kind, gentle, humble, and patient. Jesus, who lived and died for us, is the embodiment of grace. Without Him, we have no forgiveness. Without forgiveness, there is no salvation. Without salvation, everything we aspire to—success, health, and even love—is meaningless in the sense that it produces a short-lived effect. But life infused by saving grace through faith restores our souls. Combine that with fitness infused by faith, and we acquire the means to restore our bodies and press on in the hard work of being followers of Christ, spreading God's grace and having a timeless impact on the lives of others.

Perfect Grace Necessitates Perfect Justice

It's important to know that while mercy and grace are attributes of God that have been transferred to us, so also is the attribute of justice.

For God so loved the world, that he gave his only Son, that whoever believes in him should not perish but have eternal life. Whoever believes in him is not condemned, but whoever does not believe is condemned already, because he has not believed in the name of the only Son of God.

—John 3:16, 18

Justice is another characteristic that resulted from our being made in God's image. That is a concept we are very familiar with in our world today. For example, whenever a heinous crime is committed, there is a demand from society to condemn it and a response by law enforcement to correct it. We are a people of justice. As often as we can, we try to make all wrongs right and preserve proper order in a humanitarian way. This attribute we get from God, who established perfect peace. That means all of our efforts to live civilly, with virtue and goodwill, have God's fingerprints all over them.

God has instilled in us a desire to protect and serve each other. We value life and the lives of others, so we put laws in place to ensure our safety. When those laws are broken, there are consequences that have to be dealt with. In some states, the courts may impose capital punishment on murderers. This idea of retribution has its origin in God, who is our judge.

The God of peace will soon crush Satan under your feet. The grace of our Lord Jesus Christ be with you.

—Rom. 16:20

The balance of God's grace is His perfectly enforced justice. Justice keeps God from being a pushover. Sustaining perfect victory over all things is one of the main attributes of being almighty. But in order for God to be perfectly victorious, someone or something has to lose out. In this case, it is Satan, the archenemy of God. He is the perpetrator of original sin, the instigator of all idleness and everything that is gluttonous and slothful. Justice puts an end to self-indulgence. It says no to all the things that are killing our bodies and says yes to everything that is life-giving.

God Gives Grace to the Undeserved

In Chapter 1, we talked about how in the sight of God, who established good, all wrongdoing is equally offensive because it all stems from contention with Him. And because God is forever holy, He must also be forever just. He must deal with sin in a way that ensures He is forever victorious over it. Like our form of punishing the guilty, God's law says:

The wages of sin is death.

—Rom. 6:23

But God showed mercy and grace by allowing Jesus to die on the cross in our place so those who have faith in Him can be released from the just consequences.

But the free gift of God is eternal life in Christ Jesus our Lord.

—Rom. 6:23

The anatomy of grace came into being the moment God chose not to exercise capital punishment on Adam and Eve when they disobeyed Him. In their fear and shame, they stood before God, their judge, naked and afraid. God could have rightfully executed them for their lawlessness, but in His graciousness, He decided to make amends for their sins by sacrificing an animal and clothing them with its skin. That represented the very first act of pardon through immolated bloodshed.

> *And the LORD God made for Adam and for his wife garments of skins and clothed them.*
>
> —Gen. 3:21

What amazing grace! But the damage had been done. Because of their disobedience, our skin now wrinkles and blemishes over time. Our eyesight and hearing slowly fade, our hair eventually loses its color and falls out, and so do our teeth. Our youth only lasts so long before old age takes over and our bones become frail as our ability to strengthen our bodies gradually dissipates. Our metabolisms inevitably slow down, and our hearts will one day give out.

Be Sanctified in Good Health

When we make an effort to be as healthy as possible, we take a godly stance in opposition to the deteriorating effect that original sin has left on our bodies. When we eat and drink what is both lawful and helpful, we communicate to God our desire to bodily participate in being set apart and to be kept fit for every good work. This was the prayer of Jesus:

> *Sanctify them in the truth; your word is truth. As you sent me into the world, so I have sent them into the world. And for their sake I consecrate myself, that they also may be sanctified in truth.*
>
> —John 17:17–19

It was also the prayer of Paul the apostle:

Now may the God of peace himself sanctify you completely, and may your whole spirit and soul and body be kept blameless.

—1 Thess. 5:23

And it was the prayer of John the apostle:

Beloved, I pray that all may go well with you and that you may be in good health, as it goes well with your soul.

—3 John 1:2

A lot of us are under the impression that God only helps us in spiritual matters, so we rely on secular methods for fitness and are in danger of pursuing health the wrong way. We apply minimal effort to the pursuit of holiness and focus more on how we look on a cruise, by the lake, or at the beach. That attitude is quite common, and most of us can relate to it. Our concern is focused more on how we look in bikinis and board shorts, yoga pants, and muscle shirts. But where are these desires coming from? Is being healthy and having a good-looking body motivated by self-fulfillment? Each of us must examine our motivation for getting fit and in shape. I had to learn that fitness is so much more than looking good and feeling good. I thought it was about impressing each other with our attractive physiques or getting the attention and approval of others. I'd spend hours in the gym trying to impress people. I was desperately seeking acceptance, rank, and stature. I craved everyone's likes, head turns, and second looks. What that revealed was an obsession over what people thought of me and an absence of enjoyment in what God thought of me.

Attain Fitness through God's Grace

We ought to be so in love with the idea of being created in the image of God that we scripturally nourish and care for our bodies. The strength of Christ and what He accomplished with His body fits perfectly at the forefront of our minds if we'll only let it. The power of His name is more than enough to bulldoze our laziness, weakness, and self-inflicted obesity. Excessive weight gain, anorexia, and bad health in general can quickly paralyze and shackle us. In the name of Jesus, who is grace, we can break free and overcome all hindrances that prevent us from being the light of Christ.

None of us will be able to do that perfectly. But because of God's grace, all of us should strive for perfection in honor and acclaim for everything He has done. In the Bible, we find that grace is one of the most prevalent hallmarks of God's character and extends immeasurably to all His people. Grace was upon Noah during the flood, a catastrophic event in which God physically protected Noah and his family in the ark God commanded him to build.

> *Then the LORD said to Noah, "Go into the ark, you and all your household, for I have seen that you are righteous before me in this generation . . . For in seven days I will send rain on the earth forty days and forty nights, and every living thing that I have made I will blot out from the face of the ground."*
>
> —Gen. 7:1, 4

Grace was upon the people of Israel when God rescued them out of slavery in Egypt and upon Moses in the wilderness as he interceded for God's people who were prone to rebel and wander from the faith.

The LORD passed before him and proclaimed, "The LORD, the LORD, a God merciful and gracious, slow to anger, and abounding in steadfast love and faithfulness, keeping steadfast love for thousands, forgiving iniquity and transgression and sin, but who will by no means clear the guilty."

—Exod. 34:6–7

Grace was given to a lame beggar through the apostle Peter in the early days of the church. Grace made him physically strong enough to walk and jump for joy at the sight of this miraculous healing.

But Peter said, "I have no silver and gold, but what I do have I give to you. In the name of Jesus Christ of Nazareth, rise up and walk!" And he took him by the right hand and raised him up, and immediately his feet and ankles were made strong. And leaping up, he stood and began to walk . . . walking and leaping and praising God.

—Acts 3:6–9

Peter went on to testify that the author of life, Jesus, is the only one who can rightly, wholly, and irreproachably restore our bodies.

And his name—by faith in his name—has made this man strong whom you see and know, and the faith that is through Jesus has given the man this perfect health in the presence of you all.

—Acts 3:16

God's Grace Strengthens Our Bodies

The message of Jesus was that God's grace is upon all humans. It is outstretched beyond borders, for all races of people, regardless of their past or present. Jesus's death on the cross represents God's ultimate sacrifice, the pinnacle of His immeasurable grace.

In Him we have redemption through his blood, the forgiveness of our trespasses, according to the riches of his grace, which he lavished upon us, in all wisdom and insight . . . according to his purpose, which He set forth in Christ as a plan for the fullness of time, to unite all things in him, things in heaven and things on earth.

—Eph. 1:7–10

This grace was poured out to revive our souls and unify our bodies to Him. Our hearts and minds are now His. Our hands and feet belong to God, along with our voices, our eyes, our stomachs, our arms, and our legs. Every part of us has been joined and connected to Him. So this grace is available to us to provide power in our feeble conditions, being overcome by sinful cravings. When we let ourselves go, God's grace is sufficient enough to get us back on course. When we pack on the pounds in a way that's unspiritual, God's grace is made ready to motivate us for change.

Pursuing fitness through the grace of God is going to look different for everybody. It will reflect whatever His calling is for each of our lives. It will be determined through His redemptive process, through our circumstances, and through whatever He requires in equipping us for every good work. Some of us will be gifted athletes for the glory of God, others desk jockeys for the glory of God.

Some will be criminal lawyers seeking justice in the name of Christ, others doctors healing in the name of Christ. Some might be praying for God to help them build muscles, others the will and power to conquer obesity. We can presume many are going to be working hard toward lowering cholesterol and blood pressure, others battling depression and eating disorders.

The main thing to remember is that the issue doesn't start with the unhappiness that strikes us or the disappointment that sets in when looking at our bodies in the mirror. The issue starts with our attitude and condition before God. There is no one who cares more about mind, body, and soul than God. He created us, and He wants to see us healthy in every way.

If we believe in Him who is almighty, then there is no limit to what He can provide for us. No matter how overweight we are, how weak we've become, or how hopeless it may seem, we are never beyond His redemptive reach. With confidence, we should be able to look ourselves in the mirror and say, "By God's grace, I can do this!" Fitness requires hard work, commitment, and devotion. There is no one more hard working, more faithful, and more devoted than God. Fitness requires strength, endurance, and perseverance. There is no one stronger than Jesus Christ. No one has ever gained from pain more than He has, nor has anyone knuckled down in such selfless, flawless fashion to carry out God's uncanny tasks and miraculous handiwork. And there has been no greater source of empowerment, no more magnificent proxy or stout instructor than the Holy Spirit Himself.

God's Grace Sustains Our Bodies

You might ask, "What about all the extraordinary athletes who don't have faith but are healthy, fit, and prosperous in life?"

We can't deny things like good genetics, raw talent, and natural athletic ability. Yes, certain aspects of our health and fitness are affected by body type, bone structure, and DNA. We all know people who seem uncontrollably fit, and then we know those who seem uncontrollably fat. But none of that was determined by chance; it was determined by God. Your body, fat or fit, was given to you by our gracious creator. So here is the appropriate question to ask: "God, what would you have me do with the body you gave me?" There are plenty of fit and healthy people who have zero faith and rely fully on their mental toughness. But everyone believes in something. If they're not believing in God, then they're putting their belief in something else, perhaps themselves. That means they spend more time focusing on their own agendas rather than God's agenda.

We can't dispute the power of self-belief or self-will. But when you put the power of self-belief next to your belief in Christ, there is no comparison. The power of belief in Christ is immeasurable. When you put the power of self-will against the will of God, God's will always prevails. God's power is the unstoppable force that determines our destiny, and His grace is the catalyst by which it is carried out, in this life and the next.

I was once motivated by my own success and my own interests. I never really thought about the interests of God. I thought I was completely in charge of my life and could decide, all on my own, what my destiny would be. I looked to earthly things such as more exposure, fortune, and fame instead of looking to Jesus, my maker and king. I strived to be noticed, collecting trophies, stockpiling cash, and savoring the personal sensation of greatness.

Occasionally, I'd ascribe credit to someone or something other than myself, such as the military, a mentor, or an important figure in my life. Sometimes, I'd attach myself to profound quotes I lived by for inspiration. But I never brought God into the picture. It was just self-motivated taglines such as, "Never quit, never settle, and be better than the rest."

Those are good things to live by. But they're even greater in their effectiveness when the credit is ascribed to our maker. God is responsible for everyone's existence and, therefore, success. Ultimately, He is also responsible for everyone's judgment.

It is only through what's called "common grace" that God allows prosperity to be experienced by everyone. But in the end, all the trophies and medals, championships, and titles will mean nothing if they weren't achieved through saving grace—the kindness of God that exists now and into eternity. Grace enables crowned athletes to celebrate their victory in Christ and their glory in God who sustains them. Sustaining grace enables athletes to stay fit and healthy long after their glory days are over. This grace can only be found in Jesus and carried out by the Holy Spirit.

Fitness is Forged from Faith

So let's go back to that question: "God, what would you have me do with the body you gave me?" In my own life, I've gotten thinner and put on strength, grown comfortable with my figure, and then watched the thickness return and the muscles diminish from an improper diet and a short-lived workout regimen. When I worked in the fitness industry, I once entered a 60-day challenge with some of my coworkers and supervisors. I was new to the business, so I thought winning the competition would help me gain notoriety.

Sadly, that was my only intention and purpose for wanting to change my body. Long story short, I didn't win. I submitted my before-and-after pictures to the judges, but there were plenty others who had lost more fat and gained more muscle. Being in better shape did, however, help me sell more gym memberships. I felt good about myself, but it didn't last because there was no faith behind it.

My time there was all about me and what I wanted. Never once did I pray about entering the competition. Never once did I seek God in what I should eat or how I should train for it. What good were my before-and-after pics if later on there was no sustaining grace to prevent me from looking worse than before? And I did end up looking worse than before.

Too many times, I entered an unhealthy cycle of watching my weight and hitting the gym only when I absolutely had to, during the seasons of sunny skies and hot weather. But when fall and winter returned, I'd go back to the bakeries and buffets. I preferred to pursue fitness out of obligation when I was supposed to care for my body out of devotion. God wants our training to be a way of life, infused by faith, just like everything else we do.

For whatever does not proceed from faith is sin.
—Rom. 14:23

Health and fitness must be chased after with a desire for healing, both spiritually and physically, impelled by the grace of God as if mind, body, and soul are one—just like God, Jesus, and the Holy Spirit are one. Everything they do is infused with compassion and grace. Our bodies tell the story of God's monumental power in creation. The more immaculate shape we keep our bodies in, the more we exude our appreciation and gratefulness of God's creation.

Health Is Propelled by Grace

So the first step is seeing and savoring God's magnificent assembly and construction of the anatomy of grace.

The eye is the lamp of the body. So, if your eye is healthy, your whole body will be full of light.
—Matt. 6:22

Be enlightened by His word for the eternal benefit of your soul so you can embark on the journey toward a perfect body for Him, in Him, and through Him. Be delighted in His mercies that are new every morning. Begin your day with a commitment to never quit on

Him because He never quit on you—to never settle for less than the best because He will never settle for less than what's best for you.

Only by grace can we be saved from our addictions to things such as French fries and nachos, cupcakes and soda pop, beer and cigarettes. And only by grace will we be able to recover progressively with a diet and exercise plan that isn't just scientifically proven but also scripturally sound. Getting back in shape, bringing your weight down from dangerous levels, and staying healthy are all works of grace. New beginnings are made possible because grace gives us the chance to change. Unite your passions to be spiritually fit and physically fit, and be transformed by Jesus's bodily example. Lift up your eyes and cry out to the gracious father who made you, who loves you, and who nourishes you, the one who has begun a work in you that He will see to completion. Experience His freedom in fighting the good fight and overcoming bad health and sinful cravings by the power of God's grace. May we never look back, knowing that our help in times of need, in times of brokenness, pain, and despair, comes from God.

CHAPTER 8

The Good Fight of Faith

We pick and choose our battles. In middle school, I signed up to play football for the Bammel Patriots in Houston, Texas. I was totally thrilled for this opportunity. I can recall orientation day, moving through the equipment line in the gymnasium, being handed my helmet, shoulder pads, cleats, and jersey. I was burning with anticipation to make tackles, score touchdowns, and hear the crowds roar. What excited me most, though, wasn't being part of the team. It was a fact that the players got all the glory, all the fame, and all the girls.

I wondered what my next girlfriend would look like. Would she be the lead cheerleader or the valedictorian? For me, that was the start of a great life of legendary status and widespread approval. Then came the first day of practice. It was awful. We ran and ran, and then ran some more. Lifting weights was torture.

I had no idea how weak and out of shape I was as a sixth grader. I watched as other guys ran sprints much faster than I could and blasted through push-ups and pull-ups. It took me days, sometimes weeks, to learn our drills, and the playbook was way beyond my comprehension. Almost all my teammates were in better condition and had no problem catching and throwing. I ended up making the B team, the squad of last picks who clearly had less talent than the A team.

The position I wanted was wide receiver, but the coaches made me a tight end. At the start of the season, on offense, I ran my routes, blocked for others, and fulfilled my assignments. But seriously, the quarterback never looked my way, and we were winless. One day, I became completely fed up with it. During one of our home games in the second quarter, I decided it was either now or never.

I went into the huddle ready to do whatever it took. The clock was winding down, and we needed a score. Our top wide receiver jogged over from the sideline and joined us. He whispered to the quarterback what the play was, and the quarterback repeated it back to us. Once again, the play didn't involve me getting the football.

"Break!" we shouted on our way to the line of scrimmage to get set. I remember thinking I was sick of this. How long were they going to ignore me for the other guy? I was supposed to run a route in the complete opposite direction of the kid they were throwing to, a five and out. But instead, when the ball was hiked, I ran straight up the middle of the field and made my way toward the other receiver. Next thing I knew, I was wide open in position to make a play. The quarterback scrambled out of the pocket and launched the ball in the air—and it headed in my direction.

This is it! I thought to myself. This is my moment! The ball landed perfectly in my hands, and then I ran as fast as I could. The crowd roared. They cheered louder and louder the closer I got to scoring points for our team. I knew that the instant I crossed the end zone, all the long practices, stupid drills, and loud and obnoxious coaching would finally pay off. Closing in, I could see it. I could taste it. Everyone's going to be so proud of me. Dudes are going to want to be like me. It all ended about five yards too soon. One of the other team's defenders caught up to me and tackled me from behind. As I descended to the mud and grass, the ball came loose and rolled into the hands of an opposing player—a turnover—and he ran it back for a 95-yard touchdown. I couldn't believe it. I was crushed, maybe even ruined. It was probably one of the most embarrassing moments of my life. After that season, I was done with football.

Fighting the Wrong Fight

After football, I turned to other things to help me on my quest for acceptance. First, it was choir. I joined the choir to sing at competitions, hoping to gain recognition from someone in the music industry. Maybe I'd land a recording contract like New Kids on the Block did. Back then, they got all the girls. The goal, though, was to be in a band like Mötley Crüe, Poison, or Guns and Roses who seemed to have all the fun and all the money. For years, I watched Michael Jackson take the world by storm and then sit on top of it.

That's where I wanted to be, but I couldn't afford singing lessons. I had zero rhythm and really didn't possess any musical skills or even a very good voice. So I decided to do the next best thing: join a gang, of course. Now I could have high distinction and due respect through my tough, fearless persona on the wild side. As a minority, I bought into the belief that it was the white man keeping me from my place at the table. So I fought for it with anarchy, terrorizing "privileged" students, and raising hell in my classrooms. That mayhem spilled into my parents' home, the neighborhoods I grew up in, the jobs I worked at, and my relationships. It took over my life.

By the time I was a senior in high school, I decided to put my knuckle-headedness to good use in the United States Marine Corps and fight for freedom. But what I found was that the military isn't for young men without any direction or passion. It isn't for those who lack integrity or conviction, or for wild teenagers who are shallow, arrogant, and empty inside. The only thing I ended up fighting for was me. Everything was about me and what I wanted, and I'd stop at nothing to make myself happy.

The problem was the way I pursued my definition of happiness. It only brought misery, bitterness, and hostility. I was putting my faith in myself to achieve a destiny I was incapable of achieving, just like I had done in middle school. I was still looking for meaning and acceptance in all the wrong places. I hadn't learned a damn thing since junior high. I had only changed and redirected the channels through which I sought a jackpot of unending bliss.

I was stuck in a futile pursuit, fighting the wrong fight, searching for meaning in what was meaningless. My faith should have been in my maker, my lord and savior. My life should have been reflecting the image of God, bearing the fruit of the Holy Spirit, and displaying the glory of Christ. I short-circuited those things by seeking purpose and significance in the shallowness of life.

Mixed Standards Versus Fixed Standards

As a follower of Jesus, I now strive to put Him first so I can demonstrate genuine faith on a daily basis—not just at church on Sundays and not just when it's convenient. For a lot of us, as soon as we walk out the sanctuary doors, we take our spiritual glasses off and live the rest of the week with our fickle shades on. Every time we do that, we create a façade that prevents others from seeing the real us, our true selves. We create for ourselves masks—the work mask, the social mask, the spiritual mask, the family mask, and the me mask. Which one we wear depends on the people and the environment that surround us.

As a Christian man, here's what that battle looked like in the past. When I was around church people, I was on my best behavior. But as soon as I got around my drinking buddies, I consumed questionable amounts of alcohol, I talked differently, I had different mannerisms, and I filled my stomach with food that made me sick. For other people, the battle might look like a struggle with road rage or a seemingly pure relationship tainted by pre-marital sex. It could even be an under-the-radar food lover ensnared by gluttony and an appetite for destruction. Our struggles reveal that it's sometimes easy to forget the holy standard of life to which God has called us.

Abstain from every form of evil.

—1 Thess. 5:22

That's an actual verse in the Bible. We don't see it on personalized coffee cups or in people's homes as decorative apparel. Nor do we typically see it tattooed on anyone's body or even on a bumper sticker. It's because we live in this world as Christians with mixed standards based mostly on what we see rather than fixed standards based fully on what we believe. Sometimes, we act out our faith according to how we feel, not according to what God's word says. Then we look around and see others acting out their feelings and start believing that this is the norm. At first glance, it's not such a big deal. But mixed standards have caused a huge decline in the health of more than 160 million American bodies as we've become a more gluttonous nation.[2]

For years and years, I went to work to accomplish and achieve much, never once thinking about the compartmentalization of faith that is causing disparity in life. A lot of my superiors and colleagues weren't concerned about my waistline or theirs. But there were a few

---

2. Maggie Fox, "The Whole World Is Getting Fatter, New Survey Finds," *NBC News*, (May 27, 2014), https://www.nbcnews.com/better/diet-fitness/whole-world-getting-fatter-new-survey-finds-n115811.

who did, and they humbly set the example for it. When appropriate, they were kindly involved in conversation about our bodies being God's temple. Some leaders today have a meaningful, purposeful program that protects their employees from disorder and disease.

For the ones who don't, business is mostly about the pursuit of wealth and comfort. Tragically, a lot of our bosses slip further out of good physical shape yet continue thriving on and being motivated by the company's success. CEOs and board members, likewise fat and happy, flying around in private jets, eating and drinking whatever they please but still getting one day closer to retirement. All is good so long as sales are up, profits are increasing, production is rising, and the bills are getting paid. Health and fitness are easily placed on the back burner.

I would tend to take this mindset home at night. We live in a hardworking culture that has created a rat race all the way to the top. For me, at the end of a long stressful day, it was easy to become a bit weary, a little lazy, and the couch became my throne. After months and months of eating on the run, swinging by every fast-food drive-through, making very little time to exercise, it became inevitable that I gained weight and got out of shape. The only reason I could sleep at night was because I aced the self-assessment of my own standards. My spouse is good, my kids are good, the rent is paid, and there's food on the table. I'd take a look around and think, *We're doing pretty good.* Meanwhile, my body, which was at the very bottom of my priority list, was suffering internally. I didn't worry about it, though, because, again, it didn't affect what I saw or what others saw. If it ever would become an issue, I could hide my mixed standards with things like material possessions and pass them off as "blessings." If that didn't work and I still craved the appearance of doing well physically, I knew I could flee to extremes with liposuction and vain plastic surgery to remove excess fat and saggy skin. I would have had to save up money, but in the interim, I could just purchase clothes designed to slim down my figure or starve myself to maintain the approval of others.

Settling for less than God's fixed standard is the equivalent of disobedience. When we want the approval of others more than God's approval, we belittle Him. We make Him inferior instead of exalting Him as king. Our lord and savior Jesus should be our source of confidence and strength. Our only hope to fight the good fight of faith is found in Him. Every day, we enter into battles we don't need to be fighting. The battles of heart disease, cancer, anorexia, depression, and laziness—we choose to suppress them with human vices rather than conquer them with godly virtues. That is not the Christian way.

We Walk by Faith

Some of us have taken a lukewarm approach to our faith as well as our fitness, slowly but surely getting back into it. We tell stories about how we used to attend church every Sunday and were so involved, and then something bad happened. Somebody hurt us or offended us or let us down, so we quit going. We weren't getting the results we desired, so we left.

And we take this same attitude into the gym. We come up with a plan, we set a goal, we pick a training program, and then we run, we lift, we push, and we pull. We stomach the veggies and the chicken breast, the water and the rice cakes. But then we hop on that scale and don't see much of a difference, so we quit. We look in the mirror and can't see the results we desired, so we give up.

Meanwhile, everyone else is eating pizza, burgers, and hot dogs, drinking beer, wine, and margaritas without gaining a single pound. It feels like they're all doing better than we are, and everything is going right for them. They're blessed physically and spiritually; they're connecting with others, building friendships, and they don't have a single complaint. It's tough to watch, and it can lead us into fighting the wrong fight. But if we look with eyes of faith, we can stop focusing on the temporary and hone in on the timeless.

> *For we walk by faith, not by sight.*
>
> —2 Cor. 5:7

Sadly, walking by sight is a huge part of the American culture. But the people of God are meant to act in accordance with Jesus's culture, based on His authority and our acceptance of Him as lord and savior.

> *For we must all appear before the judgment seat of Christ, so that each one may receive what is due for what he has done in the body, whether good or evil.*
>
> —2 Cor. 5:10

Walking by sight gives us, mere human beings, authority over our lives. Walking by faith gives Jesus authority over our lives so God can bring out His best in us. His Holy Spirit can mature our minds, bodies, and souls to a level that goes way beyond what anyone or anything else can do. That's because everything belongs to Jesus, on earth and in heaven, in this life and the next. God has made it so. There is no place where the rule of Christ does not reach.

> *And what is this immeasurable greatness of his power toward us who believe, . . . that he worked in Christ when he raised him from the dead and seated him at his right hand in the heavenly places, far*

above all rule and authority and power and dominion, and above every name that is named, not only in this age but also in the one to come. And he put all things under his feet and gave him as head over all things to the church, which is his body, the fullness of him who fills all in all.

—Eph. 1:19–23

When we are united in Christ through faith, there is nothing or no one who can stop us or hold us back. Jesus has attained victory over all by His dynamic vigor, in His impeccable ministry, and through His bodily sacrifice. We are now the beneficiaries of His holiness, His redemption, and His grace. It all belongs to us.

So let no one boast in men. For all things are yours . . . all are yours, and you are Christ's, and Christ is God's.

—1 Cor. 3:21–23

Jesus Equips Us for the Fight

You and I live under the authority and power of Jesus. We are members of the body of Christ, a community of believers who come together in and with that same authority and power. Because of Christ, we have authority and power over death and adversities, even the heaviest weaknesses and the deepest depressions. His almighty strength is enough to vanquish our addictions, our obesity, and our sloth. His power can protect us from anything that might deter our health or keep us from a fit lifestyle, better equipping us for all kinds of ministry.

So why do we think we need something more? If we have this power living inside of us through faith, why do we look elsewhere for motivation and inspiration? We search endlessly for the perfect diet plan, for the perfect workout program, the perfect personal trainer, and the perfect gym. Some of us spend thousands of dollars a year on expensive shoes, shirts, and shorts, headbands and headphones, Fitbits, and trendy athletic gadgets. We hope for change by having all these when Christ is the only one who can provide true transformation.

When we hope in all other things, we limit the power of God in us and the power in Jesus's name through us. We transfer our faith, whether knowingly or unknowingly, to draw inspiration and power from another source, thinking it will provide higher motivation and strength. It's easy to do, and we do it quite often, but there is no such source. No other name carries greater power for change than the name of Jesus.

I wonder how many people out there are going about health and fitness all alone, unaware of the strength that Jesus provides for hope and perseverance. Doesn't it seem like everyone is kind of doing their own thing? *Look how far I've come on my own. Look at what I did. I'm doing this for me.* In almost all the social media posts you'll see, the articles you'll read, and the news stories you'll hear about, the credit either goes to the person, a new dietary supplement, or a trendy fitness program.

It seems rare to come across an article or a post about the power of God changing someone's health for the better. Very rarely will you hear a news story about the strength of Christ helping someone lose weight. That doesn't mean it's not happening; it just means no one is talking about it in that way. We keep our "religion" out of it because we think it's right to separate our spiritual activity from our physical activity. We keep our faith to ourselves because we'd rather not go there. Is it because we're afraid of what people might think? If so, it reveals a higher priority in our lives than the good news of Jesus and the great glory of God.

Neutrality Is Not the Fight

A lot of us struggle with thinking our faith is supposed to be kept hidden when we interface with others outside the walls of our churches and homes. So while we're in the gym, we put our headphones on and become introverts, not really talking to anyone. Or we'll be extroverts, talking to everyone about everything except God and our faith. I'm guilty of it. I used to talk about sports, work, and politics all the time. I went to great lengths to blend in by keeping my conversations trivial.

Instead of putting myself in a position to fight the good fight of faith, I was actually standing on the sidelines in fear of offending someone. Standing on neutral ground is not a fight. Neutrality represents the principle of tolerance and most often compromise. We cannot fear freely sharing the gospel or defending its principles on the basis of thinking it's weird or too spiritual.

The outside world is supposed to know that we stand with Christ, regardless of what they might think. They're supposed to be able to spot us anywhere, like bright lights in a dark room. Faithful Christians will peacefully yet vibrantly take Jesus everywhere they go. They want as many others as possible to know Him and be thinking of Him, not just around Christmas and Easter, and not just at weddings and funerals. Not just at church, not just at Bible study, but everywhere, including their fitness centers and gyms. Why the gym? For two reasons. One is that your faith will be tested there just like in any other context. And two is that fitness centers are a huge platform for men and women to demonstrate Christ-like qualities.

Working out and getting in shape require determination, dedication, discipline, and focus. There is no better source of those qualities than Jesus, the man who exercised them regularly throughout His ministry, even in the face of death. Staying in shape demands confidence, counterpoise, and communion. Jesus was willing to combat anything that would sabotage our efforts to remain pure and wholesome. As we take care of our bodies, we imitate Christ. He is passionate about taking care of our minds, our souls, and our bodies—spiritually and physically. His desire is for all of us to work together, constantly, to keep ourselves holy through the guidance and energy of the Holy Spirit.

> *And let steadfastness have its full effect, that you may be perfect and complete, lacking in nothing.*
> —James 1:4

God has fought the perfect fight for us, conducting the perfect evangelistic outreach to save our souls through the perfect fighter, His son Jesus Christ. God's primary concern for us has always been our hearts. He knows them better than anyone else ever will, including ourselves. He pays attention to all the things we can be oblivious to in our own lives and the lives of all others.

> *The LORD saw that the wickedness of man was great in the earth, and that every intention of the thoughts of his heart was only evil continually.*
> —Gen. 6:5

Only God has the remedy for this unhealthy, run-down condition.

> *This is the covenant that I will make with them after those days, declares the LORD: I will put my laws on their hearts, and write them on their minds . . . I will remember their sins and their lawless deeds no more.*
> —Heb. 10:16–17

Body and Strength for God's Purpose

Every one of us who is a Christian is a sinner whose heart was once continually evil but now has been saved by God's grace through faith. So, you see, every time you walk into a gym, a fitness center, a yoga studio, or a sports arena, you—your thoughts, your words, and your actions—represent Christ. For nonbelievers, their thoughts and actions are still stuck in that tragic cycle of fighting the wrong fight.

> *The fool says in his heart, "There is no God." They are corrupt, they do abominable deeds; there is none who does good.*
>
> —Ps. 14:1

Which means, no matter how hard they get after it, no matter how strong or in shape they are, no matter how friendly or charitable or gracious they may seem, their efforts are in danger of being in vain.

> *And without faith it is impossible to please him, for whoever would draw near to God must believe that he exists and that he rewards those who seek him.*
>
> —Heb. 11:6

It should sadden us to miss opportunities to share the gospel with a fellow weightlifter or a friendly jogger on the treadmill next to us, or while holding the punching bag for a fellow boxer. How quickly we forget where we came from: a fragile condition of brokenness and a complete state of darkness. Every athlete we admire and every fit guru we respect are in total darkness if they don't know God. Those hardworking people we enjoy seeing in the gym are in total darkness if they're not saved.

I understand relationships don't happen overnight. We have to build friendships from the ground up, for sure. It takes time to earn people's trust and respect. I get it. But if we're not leading the blind to sight, we could be enabling them to go into further blindness. If we're not using our health and fitness to have a positive influence on them, we might be in danger of having a negative influence on them. If we aren't displaying fitness wrapped in the glory of Christ consistently, we might be fluctuating in the fight of faith with compromise and tolerance.

It may take months or years to develop a good rapport with people or find common interests. But we must remember that the gospel is an urgent message. When dealing with nonbelievers, we must remember that eternal life and eternal death are at stake. And because we believe everything happens for a reason, we can believe God puts nonbelievers in our midst, in our gyms and fitness centers, and in our lives everywhere for a reason. So while we're at the gym, let's work out, compete, and train, hoping to purposefully reveal our savior to others. Let's exercise and care for our bodies in a way that shows our passion for Christ. Let's use our physical training in a way that pours out sweat and energy, exemplifying our value in belonging to God, our creator.

Jesus Gives Eternal Health

The foundation of our fight for fitness and the testimony of our health should be centered on the solid rock on which we stand—Jesus. Since all things have been centered on Him, it only makes sense that all things flow from Him. Since we are new creations in Him, every word spoken, every thought, every action should flow out for Him, in honor and in worship, to His praise and to His glory. Strength that lasts forever and endurance that goes the distance is built by faith rooted in Christ, with eternal health as our reward.

Every athlete exercises self-control in all things. They do it to receive a perishable wreath, but we an imperishable.

—1 Cor. 9:25

So take a stance against bad eating and the temptation to not train your body for godliness. Join the battle to help guard others' souls and to participate in the supernatural restoring of hearts and minds in all the places frequented by those struggling. Health and wellness are not something you have to take on all by yourself. Nor should you keep physical fitness separate from spiritual fitness. I used to complete a spiritual checklist for God on Sundays and then toss it away the moment I set foot in the gym, but not anymore. Now, my life in its entirety is all about Him. I want to carry Him wherever I go physically and spiritually so He can carry me through whatever I encounter physically and spiritually.

Be strong, and let us use our strength for our people and for the cities of our God, and may the LORD do what seems good to him.

—1 Chron. 19:13

Our faith belongs in Him for everything. He is the only one who will never fail us, never leave us, and never forsake us. We can devote our bodies to God, free from the fear of disappointment, and be faithful because He remains faithful. He alone is the driving force that will see us through in the good fight.

Every diet we choose, let it be surrounded prayerfully in the Holy Spirit in response to God's sovereignty, seeking to emulate the example of Jesus's body. Every weight training program or intense cardio session we take on in the gym, let it reflect the anatomy of God's grace. Let all our strength training, all our grunts and groans, replicate the blood, sweat, and tears of Christ. Let every set and every repetition be empowered by the Holy Spirit who will help us see it through. And let's sing songs to God in those moments with words like these:

When I'm fighting for my life
In a battlefield of lies
I will look into Your eyes
And I will not fear
Oh, no I will not fear

I am a Child of God
I am a chosen one
I have the power of God
And I am strong

And I won't forget
I will remember
I will believe that you are good.[3]

---

3. Jeremy Ashida, vocalist, "Child," Church Project *Volume 1*, https://open.spotify.com/album/1z5vRgacKfgCwS8bnMjSxL.

CHAPTER 9

Promise of Rewards

Every industry I've worked in, whether it was merchandise, restaurants, fitness, or construction, my customers and clients were incessantly on the lookout for discounts and free stuff. They were all inherently attracted to the promise of more for less. When I worked as a personal trainer, gym members would constantly ask if we were running any specials on training sessions. As a bar manager for some years, the busiest times in our establishment were during happy hour when the prices of alcohol and appetizers were cut in half. Even in fast food, working drive-through and front counter, we'd have cars wrapped around the building and lines of hungry people out the door on "Free Breakfast Day."

For decades, mailboxes have gotten stuffed with more and more coupons—buy one, get one free and zero percent interest on credit cards. Nowadays, most grocery stores have some type of rewards program, and retail stores give bonus points for future purchases. There is a competitive war going on, a fight to secure sales and revenue today, tomorrow, and for the future. Businesses are forced to broadcast savings galore if they hope to survive.

Our Idea of Rewards Is Distorted

The world wasn't always like this. There was a time when everything in it was free. No one had to barter or beg, and there was no negotiating or haggling. There was no such thing as financial pressure, anxiety over costs and expenses, or stress over profits and losses. In the beginning, God freely gave everything by filling the earth for us with food, water, and shelter. All that He asked was for us to give back to Him in the form of obedience, to reflect His glory, and to be united with Him in purpose by growing together and giving each other knowledge, instruction, love, support, and nourishment.

> *So God created man in his own image, in the image of God he created him; male and female . . . And God blessed them. And God said to them, "Be fruitful and multiply and fill the earth and subdue it, and have dominion over the fish . . . over every living thing . . . and every tree with seed in its fruit. You shall have them for food."*
>
> —Gen. 1:27–29

In the beginning, there was no need for rewards. To be created by God, to be given life, and to be in relationship with Him was its own reward. He was our equity, our profit, our treasure, and our good deposit. He alone was our reward, and that is still true today. But the difference now is this tension that exists as we find it easier to live for other things such as possessions and money. For some of us, the struggle continues deeper into various forms of vanity, self-worship, and the idolization of a wealthy lifestyle.

My heart used to pull for the flesh in the tug of war with the spirit over what I truly valued. Life had become a game, and the clock was ticking, so I played hard and played to win. During the week, I'd hustle to survive, banging away toward that promotion, anxious to move up in the world. On the weekends, I'd reward myself.

My focus shifted to simple pleasures, pampering and leisure, loafing and lounging. I'd post pictures on social media, broadcasting how great my achievements were because I worked so hard. I'd tweet highly energized quotes that defined my earned success. I wanted everyone to know what a great time I was having, that my days and nights were thrilling with endless entertainment.

Before I was a Christian, I had adopted a common misbelief called karma. It's a belief that if we do good deeds, only good things will happen to us in return, and we'll do well and live happy lives. Karma is most often accepted by people who fear doing bad things for the simple reason that they don't want anything bad to happen to them. I mistakenly believed that what goes around comes around and never wanted to be associated with suffering, loss, or rejection. I thought getting rejected was a sign of weakness and that suffering meant I clearly messed up or did something wrong.

We Need a Redefinition of Rewards

Our idea of how rewards work and how they're attained is defined for the most part by our culture. If we were to drive through a rich neighborhood filled with country club golf courses, big mansions, nice cars in the driveways, and pools in the backyards, we'd think the residents there had it all figured out. Without even meeting them, we'd probably conclude they deserved to get to where they are. But if we were to take a stroll into the ghetto where there are homeless people begging for change, we'd think they must have screwed up royally for being so poor.

I'll be the first to admit, I don't want to be poor. I hate being broke. I hate not knowing where my next meal is going to come from, and I loathe the thought of getting kicked out of my home with my family on the streets. I know what it's like to have zero dollars in my checking account and zero funds in savings. In the past, I'd work 50 hours per week just to watch my paycheck go bye-bye to bills past due. I've been down before, and it's depressing. I've taken money from my own kids' piggy banks to buy groceries. I hated that that's what it came to.

So what did I do after that embarrassing experience? I did everything in my power to keep it from happening again. If that meant I was working on Sunday when church was going on, so be it. If it meant I couldn't make time for diet and exercise, I didn't care. I took control of the situation the best way I knew how, through dogged persistence and self-determination.

Constantly, my focus was on working long shifts, putting in the hours, saving, and cutting back, which meant no more donations and no more giving to the church. But the problem with the ideology of safeguarding my own future was that it took the place of my theology, which led me to deny Jesus as lord over my financial peace and security. And because I could no longer participate in anything spiritually good or physically beneficial, my mind, soul, and body paid the price.

Rewards Must Be Defined Biblically

The book of Job in the Bible reminds us that it is God who has sovereign control over blessings and rewards. It tells us that even through hard times, heartbreak, and harrowing circumstances, God is extraordinarily faithful to those who are relentlessly devoted to Him.

Have you considered my servant Job, that there is none like him on the earth, a blameless and upright man, who fears God and turns away from evil?

—Job 1:8

What an awesome statement for God to make about one of His beloved children! I pray that one day God can say the same about me. Job was a righteous and moral man, virtuous, above reproach, and he honored God with his life and body. Job was blessed beyond belief, extremely wealthy and successful. He had plenty of friends and a great family, and he was a charitable contributor and longstanding member of high society. But one day the devil challenged God saying this:

> *Have you not put a hedge around him and his house and all that he has, on every side? You have blessed the work of his hands, and his possessions have increased in the land. But stretch out your hand and touch all that he has, and he will curse you to your face.*
>
> —Job 1:10–11

The depth of God's relationship with Job was far more profound than rewards for good behavior and prosperity for religious devotion. So He allowed Satan to test Job by taking away all that was dear to him. And in a moment's time, Job lost everything. His kids were suddenly deceased, his assets and real estate destroyed, and all his prized possessions gone. He was a guy who had everything a man ever dreamed of, and now he was left homeless, hapless, and helpless. But because he had a godly definition of rewards through faith, his response was pious and worshipful.

> *"The LORD gave, and the LORD has taken away; blessed be the name of the LORD." In all this Job did not sin or charge God with wrong.*
>
> —Job 1:21–22

Satan's challenge then went even further with an attack on Job's body and health.

So Satan . . . struck Job with loathsome sores from the sole of his foot to the crown of his head. And he took a piece of broken pottery with which to scrape himself while he sat in the ashes.

—Job 2:7–8

It wasn't until Job's skin and bones ached with severe unending pain that he began to wonder why this was happening to him. In short, he questioned God, he pleaded with God, and he even complained to God, but he never lost sight of his commitment to God. Job was confused about why he had to suffer so much, but through all the misery, he realized that none of us is ever in a position to question God's authority over our physical lives.

I know that you can do all things, and that no purpose of yours can be thwarted. . . . Therefore I have uttered what I did not understand, things too wonderful for me, which I did not know . . . but now my eyes see you; therefore I despise myself and repent.

—Job 42:1–3, 5–6

Even though Job didn't think he deserved what happened to him, he dealt with it by faith, trusting in God's promises and mighty ways. God in His sovereignty allows affliction in the world for the grand purposes of His glory, but He also rewards for the same reason. In this case, Job was afflicted and put to the test but also rewarded for his humility and steadfastness. Life handed him some serious lemons, and then the Lord provided him with an abundance of lemonade. In the end, Job came out on the other side, stronger, healthier, and truly transformed.

And the LORD restored the fortunes of Job, when he had prayed. . . . And the LORD gave Job twice as much as he had before. . . . And the LORD

blessed the latter days of Job more than his beginning. . . . And after this
Job lived 140 years, and saw his sons, and his sons' sons, four generations.
—Job 42:10, 12, 16

Only God Provides Ultimate Health and Fitness

For the longest time, I lived with this notion that I was entitled to rewards, so I became a go-getter in that sense. I thought God wasn't able to get me a big enough house or a nice enough car and that He was too limited to provide any kind of financial security for me. And because of the amount of suffering that can be associated with poverty, I developed the attitude that if I didn't take care of myself, no one would.

So my body got stuck in the middle as God sought to draw me near to Him, but my mouth only hungered and thirsted for relaxation and riches. My eyes wandered toward fantasies and success. That was part of my problem. I was very fixated on everything I could physically see. I assumed that because I couldn't see God, He was incapable of being part of my physical solutions.

When an attack on our bodies or our health comes along, like it did with Job, it seems that the first thing we want to do is blame God. Or perhaps if we've become unhappy with how we look and dissatisfied with how we were created, we almost immediately turn our backs on our creator. Lanky legs, chubby cheeks, small arms, and tiny chests can make us think God gave us the short end of the stick. That's why when it comes to physical fitness, so many of us place our faith and hope in tangible maneuvers to shed fat, build muscle, and get in shape. We tell ourselves we don't need God, so we turn to science and nature, biochemistry and physiology, forgetting that God is the one who rewarded us with that knowledge and information.

We seem to be far more interested in listening to a famous doctor boycott carbs and fats or a celebrity bodybuilder praising egg whites and lean beef. We're so much more drawn to the hype of it all that we just drink whatever supplement is most popular and take whatever pills are trending. The reason is that what we see all around us are weight loss products, advertisements for cutting-edge diet plans, and exercise machines that say they can guarantee us results. Automatically, we're drawn to those things. We feed off the expert nutrition tips and secret formulas, simply due to the power of marketing and hard-sell persuasion.

But when considering physical wellness products, it's important to know which companies are out to scam us and which ones are actually legitimate. Whichever ones you purchase, make sure to do extensive research prior to making a commitment. And remember to pray about it. Seek the Lord in it, as only He can provide ultimate health and fitness.

Before I decided to use AdvoCare products to help me train, I was happy to find that their number-one guiding principle for success is to honor God. Organizations like that have their products tested for purity. They commit to responsible nutrition and want all consumers to make informed decisions about what they put into their bodies. AdvoCare understands that the purpose of health and fitness is bigger than themselves, so they give back through their foundation and share a great testimony with the rest of God's world.

Rewards Aren't Meant to be Self-Serving

There is a deeper meaning to nutrition and supplements that I didn't always get. I would mindlessly buy pills and powders to get results. A lot of us purchase plans, programs, videos, and equipment to produce the "new you." But somewhere between 65 percent and 80 percent of people who lose weight gain it all back and then some. Eight out of 10 people end up worse off than they started.

Truth be told, there are some fast, effective weight loss products out there. I have personally improved my body through online products, diets, and popular workout routines. But regardless of what I tried or what I put myself through physically, I never found a way to avoid or prevent relapse—because what I needed and what I wanted were two very different things.

What I wanted was to look better naked. The promise of my rewards was centered on being more physically attractive to enhance my pursuit of acceptance and affirmation. What I desired was for everyone to want to take a picture with me, like a celebrity, making memories with my hot, handsome self. What I wanted was to always be the center of attention and be the most important person everywhere I went. Alongside me was my hot, female bride. We'd be each other's trophies to ensure we both prospered and achieved all we wanted. That was the fairy tale I believed in while pumping iron and doing cardio every single day for years.

What I needed was to remember that my body is not my own. I was focused on working hard toward a life that would produce happiness, with me as the center and God as a mere spotter, only calling for His help when the weightiness of life got too heavy. I had forgotten that my body belongs to Him.

> *I have been crucified with Christ. It is no longer I who live, but Christ who lives in me. And the life I now live in the flesh I live by faith in the Son of God, who loved me and gave himself for me.*
>
> —Gal. 2:20

What I needed was to remember that my "new you" is already in Christ and that fighting the good fight is a work of faith, not a work of self-confidence. His promise of rewards is far more than I could ever attain on my own.

> *"Do not work for the food that perishes, but for the food that endures to eternal life, which the Son of Man will give to you. For on him God the Father has set his seal." Then they said to him, "What must we do, to be doing the works of God?" Jesus answered them, "This is the work of God, that you believe in him whom he has sent."*
>
> —John 6:27–29

What I needed was to remember that His rewards are full-bodied and plentiful, overflowing in this life and the next.

> *Come, everyone who thirsts, come to the waters; and he who has no money, come, buy and eat! Come, buy wine and milk without money and without price. Why do you spend your money for that which is not bread, and your labor for that which does not satisfy? Listen diligently to me, and eat what is good, and delight yourselves in rich food. Incline your ear, and come to me; hear, that your soul may live; and I will make with you an everlasting covenant.*
>
> —Isa. 55:1–3

Faith-Infused Health and Fitness

God promises that when we align our physical appetites with our spiritual appetites and submit them both to Him, we set ourselves up even more to receive God's earthly rewards, as well as His eternal rewards. When we allow Him to speak to us on physical matters, our good health produces a personally refined clarity to gain wisdom on how we must feed our souls and how we must feed our bodies, which are His temple. When our bodies serve as physical evidence that our minds are focused on the promise of heavenly rewards, it reveals that we are in the fight, battling against sinful cravings and taking up our cross to follow Him.

I press on toward the goal for the prize of the upward call of God in Christ Jesus.

—Phil. 3:14

You see, our fitness goals should be in response to the upward call. Goals, no matter how personal, should never be centered on what our hearts and bodies naturally desire. This was very difficult for me to do, even as a believer. I never once prayed or asked God what plans He had for my body. I seldom sought His counsel for moderation in what I ate or drank. This is a mistake that is easy for all believers to make. When we don't protect our bodies from falling short in that area, it quickly becomes obvious to those around us. We must educate each other and keep each other accountable.

Brothers, join in imitating me, and keep your eyes on those who walk according to the example you have in us. For many, of whom I have often told you and now tell you even with tears, walk as enemies of the cross of Christ. Their end is destruction, their god is their belly, and they glory in their shame, with minds set on earthly things. But our citizenship is in heaven, and from it we await a Savior, the Lord Jesus Christ, who will transform our lowly body to be like his glorious body.

—Phil. 3:17–21

In the same way we protect our minds from spiritual and moral downfall, we must be careful and live healthily to shield our bodies from physical downfall. Since we now know that our bodies are a dwelling place for God's spirit, let us ask ourselves if this is important to us. Do we want to hear from God on physical matters or only spiritual? Is our faith distorted if we only make Jesus lord over our spiritual pursuits and not our physical ones? The Bible encourages us to unite all areas of our life under Him.

And whatever you do, in word or deed, do everything in the name of the Lord Jesus, giving thanks to God the Father through him.

—Col. 3:17

The Gift of Faith Overcomes Physically

Doing everything in the name of Jesus prevents us from taking advantage of our freedom in Christ by eating and drinking whatever we please. Although it might seem harmless, history has shown that rewarding our bodies constantly with high-sugar processed snacks such as cupcakes, cookies, and other junk inevitably becomes dangerous to our health. Since the 1970s, the rise in Type 2 diabetes, for example, has caused a staggering increase in the need for insulin treatment nationwide.[4] It's not just adults, either.

Our kids are having metabolic meltdowns. The number of obese children has gone up significantly over the last three decades. Today, processed foods make up more than 60 percent of our diets. The average American will consume about 29 pounds of French fries, 23 pounds of pizza, 24 pounds of ice cream, and about 53 gallons of soda each year.

Factor in social drinking, nightcaps, and the occasional cigarette, and the chances of our arteries remaining unclogged aren't in our favor. The more we clog our arteries, the higher the risk of having a full-blown heart attack or stroke. The symptoms of a stroke include

---

4. "Long-Term Trends in Diabetes," *CDC's Division of Diabetes Translation*, (April 2017), https://www.cdc.gov/diabetes/statistics/slides/long_term_trends.pdf.

vertigo, paralysis, mental confusion, speech loss, and blurred vision. All these could potentially put us at a physical disadvantage that, in turn, could have a negative effect on our ministries and our missions.

I believe we shouldn't sell ourselves short for temporary rewards that life has to offer if they're attached to diseases, disorders, and impairment of judgment. When we commit to God both physically and spiritually, the windows of heaven are opened to pour down on us power and strength, the same power and strength Jesus used to defeat physical death.

> *For everyone who has been born of God overcomes the world. And this is the victory that has overcome the world—our faith. Who is it that overcomes the world except the one who believes that Jesus is the Son of God?*
> —1 John 5:4–5

We need that same power and strength to conquer obesity, anorexia, diabetes, and anything else that is currently killing us. We need to be desperate for that same power and strength in times of depression and laziness. Whenever we experience a lack of confidence or a deficiency in motivation, we should run to the cross of Christ. Jesus is the food that endures, the Bread of Life that perseveres. He freely gives Himself to us to fill all the empty voids in our hearts, our minds, our souls, and our bodies. He promises to set us free from all pain and hurt, two of life's stumbling blocks that can cripple our health, our ministry, and our witness.

> *They shall hunger no more, neither thirst anymore; the sun shall not strike them, nor any scorching heat. For the Lamb in the midst of the throne will be their shepherd, and he will guide them to springs of living water, and God will wipe away every tear from their eyes.*
> —Rev. 7:16–17

Live for the True Rewards

The moment I stopped chasing after the rewards of this world, I knew I needed to do it with others. Collectively, we should possess a healthy fear of God in our hearts and minds that is reverent throughout all our bodies and evident in our diet and exercise. This is for the benefit of followers of Jesus who are set apart by God, but also for the benefit of the church. Our families, our loved ones, our children—what good are we doing each other if we just overeat and overdrink when we get together? What kind of example are we setting for our kids? What are we teaching them about the posture to attain rewards?

Demonstrating Christ-likeness through our physical fitness is one way we can help build up the church. It's a celebration of His rewards that opens doors to sharing the gospel and providing pathways to edify others. For all Christians, ensuring the tireless demonstration of Christ-likeness in everything we do is part of who we are. It's our ministry; it is our calling.

And let us not grow weary of doing good, for in due season we will reap, if we do not give up. So then, as we have the opportunity, let us do good to everyone, and especially to those who are of the household of faith.
—Gal. 6:9–10

Eating and drinking in moderation, strict diet and strenuous exercise—it's all tough. It's a lot easier said than done. But when we do it all for God and His glory, we can testify of Him as our only inspiration and success. When we do it in God's strength together as the body of Christ, we affirm we aren't living for food alone but by every word that proceeds from His mouth. When we submit to the authority of scripture, we affirm our belief in its authenticity and power.

*All Scripture is breathed out by God and profitable for teaching . . .
and for training in righteousness, that the man of God may be complete, equipped for every good work.*

—2 Tim. 3:16–17

God's Words are Priceless Rewards

I used to treat God's word as if it were just a boring old encyclope-
dia. I thought it was a long, drawn-out rule book for spiritual types
who wouldn't know how to behave or enjoy life without religious
practice. I used to be convinced that genuine peace of mind came
solely from within and that we don't need God's laws or commands.
I thought true rewards were found detached from God in self-dis-
covery on solo road trips, vacations, nature hikes, and so forth.
While all of those things are fun and good, what I missed was that
behind every earthly commandment of God, is a heavenly promise
from God.

The scriptures are a detailed schematic of deliverance, the blueprint for victory, and the treasure map that leads to endless riches
found in Jesus. Within every temporary requirement of God, therein
lies an eternal reward from God. In all the days of the prophets, we
see God fulfilling His promises with great rewards, preparing our
hearts for His greatest promise and most awesome reward—our
savior. On the night Jesus was betrayed, He said this:

*Do you think that I cannot appeal to my Father, and he will at once
send me more than twelve legions of angels? But how then should the
Scriptures be fulfilled, that it must be so? . . . But all this has taken place
that the Scriptures of the prophets might be fulfilled.*

—Matt. 26:53–54, 56

Every day of Jesus's life and ministry was a fulfillment of God's word. Everything He went through was to ensure that not even one of God's promises would be broken and to guarantee us access to His rewards. How beautiful it is to read about Jesus's bravery for God and His passion to be the handiwork of God. How beautiful it is, now that we are His handiwork, when we can hold up a mirror to our own lives and see scripture fulfilled in how we train for godliness and bear good fruit as healthy trees. How wonderful He is to us who stand firm on His word all the days of our lives.

> *Therefore do not throw away your confidence, which has a great reward. For you have need of endurance, so that when you have done the will of God you may receive what is promised.*
>
> —Heb. 10:35–36

There is a right way to revel in goodness, a true form of living long and prospering, feasting on timeless gifts. It's through the hard work and obedience involved in trusting God with everything, in everything, and for everything. When we lay down our lives and make sacrifices for Him, He always comes through for us with priceless blessings.

> *Blessed is everyone who fears the LORD, who walks in his ways! You shall eat the fruit of the labor of your hands; you shall be blessed, and it shall be well with you. Your wife will be like a fruitful vine within your house; your children will be like olive shoots around your table. Behold, thus shall the man be blessed who fears the LORD. The LORD bless you from Zion! May you see the prosperity of Jerusalem all the days of your life! May you see your children's children! Peace be upon Israel!*
>
> —Ps. 128

Use Your Body in a Gospel-Centered Way

There is a right way to pursue rewards, and it's through the motivation of the gospel, the good news that Christ died for our sins. While His blood that He shed on the cross covered my gluttony and lack of self-control, it was no excuse for me to live in a sloppy manner. I had to look to Him for diet, discipline, and diligence. He died for my drunkenness, and by His power, I learned how to drink in moderation. He died for my bulimia so that by His grace I could stop binge eating.

By His mercy, I stopped making myself throw up and chose Jesus over junk food. He died for my steroid abuse. He was there to help me put the needle down and instead inject the Holy Spirit into my body. He died for all our secret sins, and He'll be here to help us break the silence in the midst of all these broken, empty promises.

Jesus will be there the next time you're in the gym. Even if it seems like you're the fattest, slowest, weakest individual lifting weights in a puddle of your own sweat, know that the faithful stewarding of your body here on earth produces rewards in heaven. Invite Him into all your workouts, your jogs, your hikes, all your physical activity. Let your highest climbs and biggest struggles be dominated by His ever-increasing power. Our savior is never going away, and in fact, He promises to return for us.

> *Yes, we are of good courage, and we would rather be away from the body and at home with the Lord. So whether we are at home or away, we make it our aim to please him.*
>
> —2 Cor. 5:8–9

Just as He did with Job, our God will see us through from every starting point to every finish line. Of all the possible ways to pursue health and fitness, make it your aim to please God by choosing the way that will best represent His strength and His image. If you've gotten into terrible shape and need to change some unhealthy ways, make it your aim to please Him by praying for healthy direction and physical guidance. If you're ever in the doctor's office with sad news of a disease or disorder that is robbing you of comfort and hope, make it your aim to please God by allowing Him to guide you in the fight for your life.

If you're overwhelmed with the busyness of life, pray and ask Jesus what you can eat if you have to grab fast food on the run. If you frequently have work obligations that require you to dine out or be social for clients and guests, remember that you are an ambassador for Christ, first and foremost. Every day before breakfast, lunch, and dinner, let Jesus guide you into healthy food choices for the nourishment of your body. At home, pray about what to feed your families. Let the Holy Spirit be involved in the clipping of coupons, the savings, and the grocery store runs.

And never forget that we chose this struggle. We chose this way of life. It dates all the way back to the beginning when Adam and Eve partook of the forbidden fruit that wasn't for sale, and it cost them everything. We chose the struggle, but Jesus paid for it all. He restores the days of old with a new promise and invites us into holy matrimony with Him, forever and ever. Amen.

The Spirit and the Bride say, "Come." And let the one who hears say, "Come." And let the one who is thirsty come; let the one who desires take the water of life without price.

—Rev. 22:17

CHAPTER 10

Build on the Rock

God wired me for victory. I often dream of long-lasting victory and never-ending success. I don't particularly enjoy losing or failing. It's never what I strive for. I always want to do my best, be the best, and celebrate in the best way. There is an exhilaration that I desire to experience as a winner, a titleholder, and a conqueror. When I win, I encounter an extraordinary feeling of happiness that makes life worth living.

I've also fantasized about glory, legacy, and greatness. Being the center of attention or in the spotlight and getting my 15 minutes of fame was something I aspired to in the past. When I hear crowds cheer the moment their favorite baseball player smashes a home run to win the World Series, it's the thrill I wish I could give to the fans someday. When a famous basketball player drains a last-second three-pointer from mid-court for the championship and every spectator goes wild, that's a triumph I'd love to experience firsthand.

Whether it's crossing the finish line first, scoring the game-winning touchdown, competing for Olympic gold, or knocking out a fierce opponent, most of us seek the intense pleasure and satisfaction of being victorious. Whether we realize it or not, we are all wired for victory. We are naturally goal setters, challenge takers, and mission accomplishers. That's because we were made in the image of God, who overcomes all things and is victorious in all things. His word declares Him the greatest champion heaven and earth have ever seen.

O Lord, our Lord, how majestic is your name in all the earth! You have set your glory above the heavens. Out of the mouth of babies and infants, you have established strength because of your foes, to still the enemy and the avenger. When I look at your heavens, the work of your fingers, the moon and the stars, which you have set in place, what is man that you are mindful of him, and the son of man that you care for him?

—Ps. 8:1–4

However, as much as we aspire to be like our role models and heroes or imagine how great success can be, God is higher than them all and the most successful. He demonstrates that in everything He does by His incomparable wisdom and perfect strength. Whatever our situation is, God's desire is for us to look upward and pursue Him so He can give victory over difficulty to us all.

Yet you have made him a little lower than the heavenly beings and crowned him with glory and honor. You have given him dominion over the works of your hands; you have put all things under his feet, all sheep and oxen, and also the beasts of the field, the birds of the heavens, and the fish of the sea, whatever passes along the paths of the seas. O Lord, our Lord, how majestic is your name in all the earth!

—Ps. 8:5–9

God is the foundation on which life's success is built. God is where success begins and ends. As Psalm 8 tells us, we are overcomers through Him. We can be victorious because of His great victory and majesty. Knowing that, we can conclude that personal success was never meant to be experienced apart from our maker.

Stepping Out of Bounds

Achievement was never meant to be void of God or outside His glory. As the creator of earth and the originator of all humankind, God wants us to learn His ways and His word so we can live and work according to His definition of achievement and success. So many times I've tried to define winning as getting ahead on my own, but I only set myself back and set myself up for massive failure. My motives were tarnished with impropriety and greed.

When I lacked character, it caused me and others to shift since we'd stop at nothing to get our own way. I misplaced integrity, discipline, and genuine leadership for the envious number one, the top prize, and the cream of the crop. I lied, cheated, scammed, and deceived to get far in life, but because I lacked character, it all inevitably came crashing down. God's word warns us about such dishonesty and decadence.

> *Therefore this iniquity shall be to you like a breach in a high wall, bulging out and about to collapse, whose breaking comes suddenly, in an instant; and its breaking is like that of a potter's vessel that is smashed so ruthlessly that among its fragments not a shard is found with which to take fire from the hearth, or to dig up water out of the cistern.*
> —Isa. 30:13–14

It seems like every arena of society has been stained with unforgettable fallouts and scandals. From sports athletes' doping to the film industry's sexual misconduct and abuse, no amount of money, not even millions of dollars, can protect us from shame or disgrace. From perverse politicians to corrupt public officials, we're so off track that this stuff even affects our kids' schools. It infectiously creeps its way into our neighborhoods, our homes, and our communities. What's the issue?

I can't speak for anyone else, but the core of my issue was arrogance. My rise and fall to nothing was because of a spiritually weak foundation. Even though I knew I shouldn't have been careless with my life, I did it anyway. In my pride, I disregarded the commands of my maker and ignored the wise counsel of my savior. But God, in His mercy, opened my eyes and ears to finally pay close attention to what He was saying.

> *Everyone then who hears these words of mine and does them will be like a wise man who built his house on the rock. And the rain fell, and the floods came, and the winds blew and beat on that house, but it did not fall, because it has been founded on the rock. And everyone who hears these words of mine and does not do them will be like a foolish man who built his house on the sand. And the rain fell, and the floods came, and the winds blew and beat against that house, and it fell, and great was the fall of it.*
>
> —Matt. 7:24–27

God's Word Is Our Foundation for Strength

If you're like me, you've struggled with the words of the Bible. You've probably thought the words of God, the prophets, Jesus, and the apostles are far-fetched and outdated for our generation. We would rather have something fresh, fast, and flamboyant. We want advice that's not so rigid and narrow-minded. I wanted a doctrine that could help me establish my own little comfort zone, positioned for life at ease where the bending and breaking of rules was tolerated. But what I had to be reminded of was that God's words are timeless principles on which I can stand firm today, tomorrow, and forever.

God's word is applicable for everyone, for every age, no matter the time period or stage of life we're in. When it comes to our body's health and fitness, God's word and ways have the power to overcome any condition, any shape, in the sense that it provides eternal healing for eternal life. That is why we must build our bodies on the rock—Jesus. Psalm 1 tells us that physically healthy and spiritually fit are the people who build their lives on God's word.

He is like a tree planted by streams of water that yields its fruit in its season, and its leaf does not wither.

—Ps. 1:3

According to Jesus, only good trees can bear good fruit, and the bad ones bear bad fruit. We either establish ourselves on the firm footing of God's teaching or ignore Him and be swallowed up by quicksand. We have a choice to make, and none of us is exempt. Whether you've been fit your whole life without God or fat your whole life with God, everyone who is in Christ has a calling to mobilize themselves and others toward all-out ministry.

As each has received a gift, use it to serve one another, as good stewards of God's varied grace . . . whoever serves, as one who serves by the strength that God supplies—in order that in everything God may be glorified through Jesus Christ. To him belong glory and dominion forever and ever. Amen.

—1 Pet. 4:10–11

God has given each of us the tools to succeed at our own level, wherever we are on the weight scale and whatever our condition or circumstance calls for. Remember, no matter what our limitations might be or how terrible our eating habits have become, our bodies are never beyond the redemptive reach of Jesus. Fitness isn't just for the super athletic and the ones who love doing it. Building your body on the rock so God can be glorified in everything includes everyone from all walks of life—our youth, the elderly, moms and dads, amputees, the handicapped, the chronically ill, the obese, the morbidly obese, the super morbidly obese, the skinnies, and the anorexic. Exceptions are not excuses.

Be Spiritually and Physically Fit

You could be the fittest person on the planet with the fastest metabolism science has ever seen, but without Jesus, without listening to His words, you have no advantage past the point of death.

> *It is the Spirit who gives life; the flesh is no help at all. The words that I have spoken to you are spirit and life.*
>
> —John 6:63

Jesus informs us that the body was never meant to be enhanced and strengthened at the expense of one's soul. The body and soul go hand in hand, but our souls are always the higher priority. When we take a look at the ministry of Jesus, His focus and His motivation are, without a doubt, heavenly. But even He needed to be physically healthy for everything God called Him to do. While Jesus was in the flesh, His primary concern pertained to our getting right with God spiritually. However, the moment faith comes to fruition, everything about us physically must get right with Him as well so we can live out the kingdom of God that has burst into power and reality for us, even now, here on earth.

> *My son, do not forget my teaching, but let your heart keep my commandments, for length of days and years of life and peace they will add to you.*
>
> —Prov. 3:1–2

Our supernatural assignment involves our physical health. When we change our diet and exercise based on what God speaks to us, the hunger pains of denying unhealthy food and the soreness from rigorous training produce a concord through which He can provide a fullness for vitality. Whenever we abstain from gluttonous ways for the sake of the kingdom to incorporate healthy eating habits, there is an earthly blessing that God bestows on us, as well as a peculiar glory and honor waiting for us in heaven.

Putting off laziness for the sake of the gospel and putting on the energy of the Holy Spirit guides us into meaningful health and purposeful strength that lasts an entire lifetime and into eternity. Maintaining the mindset of Jesus strengthens our faith and forges an ironclad perseverance for fitness.

Since therefore Christ suffered in the flesh, arm yourselves with the same way of thinking, for whoever has suffered in the flesh has ceased from sin, so as to live for the rest of the time in the flesh no longer for human passions but for the will of God.

—1 Pet. 4:1–2

God is the Greatest of All Time

Throughout history, there have been many greats—the greatest champions, the greatest athletes, the greatest players, the greatest victors, the greatest kings and queens, the greatest conquerors. But none of them compare to the greatness of our God. Yes, so many have gained legendary status by achieving great things. We admire their medals, their titles, and their trophies, but only Jesus possesses an eternal dynasty.

Only Jesus, who demonstrates unmatchable power and strength by conquering death, provides victory that no one else can promise. No amount of human skill, mastery, or craftsmanship could ever defeat the grave. No team of engineers, scientists, or doctors will ever be able to overcome death. The biggest win, the most awe-inspiring championship was attained by Jesus Christ on the cross.

He is our example, our model, for the importance of training our bodies to be physically ready. Jesus's path to accomplishing His work was definitely a strenuous one. He traveled everywhere on land by foot, speaking daily to big crowds with authority and enthusiasm. He climbed mountains, hiked up steep hills, and woke up early to get on His knees and pray.

Healing the sick, reviving the lifeless—it all required His energy. And then He was brutally beaten and endured severe torture before bearing His own cross and being nailed to it on His hands and feet. Jesus was crucified, but for the win. He prevailed with His own body and His own blood. The body of Christ was given up for us in love to subdue our hate. His blood was shed for us in strength to overcome our weakness. His body was given to us with power, His blood with life. What better way to build your body on the rock than through His sacrificial love and a life that overcame death with unlimited power and unbeatable strength. There is no better way than to follow His instruction and emulate His example.

So how do we do that? We lay everything down at His feet, remembering that for every barrier, every obstacle, and every struggle, God has provided a way to overcome in Jesus. All our goals and dreams can be attained as long as they extend from the firm foundation of Jesus's strength. Through pillars of truth and biblically prescribed techniques, we can strive to achieve godly health and godly fitness.

The First Step to Building on the Rock

Faith-infused fitness begins with fasting and prayer. Giving up food and time to get on our knees to talk to God is a sincere physical demonstration of longing for God's help. Seeking His help enables us to build character so we can build on the rock. Character is our key ingredient, the pre-workout, so to speak, for a strong foundation of godly health and fitness.

Character is the seed planted in us to yield good fruit. With it, we prevent rotten schemes and decaying scams so there's no cracks in our groundwork. Character allows us to look inside our own hearts so the truth about who we really are can surface.

> *Examine yourselves, to see whether you are in the faith. Test yourselves. Or do you not realize this about yourselves, that Jesus Christ is in you?—unless indeed you fail to meet the test!*
>
> —2 Cor. 13:5

This is an important scripture for all of us to fast and pray over. Everyone who calls themselves a Christian should confirm they are of the faith and should know without a doubt that Jesus Christ is in them. In order to live for Him in every way, He must encompass our whole being, from top to bottom. Once we have assurance of faith, we can begin to inquire of God about the necessary changes we must make to build our bodies for Him.

For some of us, those changes might be a few minor tweaks here and there. For the rest of us, it will be a major resurgence, a huge awakening and culture shock. It's going to be difficult. It will require coming to grips with God and others about every area of our lives, even the private matters, the ones we are careful not to expose. But before we do anything, there are three practical areas we should begin to fast and pray about: our time, our tendencies, and our treasure.

Make Time for Your Body

Most people's bodily training and exercise are built around their work schedules. My wife and I both have jobs, so we designed a 30-minute program that fits our timetable without interrupting prior commitments or daily responsibilities. We usually hit the gym right after the kids get out of school. In some ways, it's a family occasion so our children can see firsthand that Mom and Dad value gym time. There are also plenty of days when we can't make it, so we exercise in the comfort of our own home. This is fun because the kids enjoy participating in cardio and bodyweight conditioning.

You see, we make time for it because we believe that faith-infused training is one way to honor God with our bodies. We believe it aligns with scripture and the biblical qualities that characterize the Christian walk. Peter the apostle teaches us about supplementing our faith with virtues (2 Pet. 1:5–9). These virtues, things like self-control, endurance, diligence, discipline, steadfastness, family love, and affection, apply spiritually and physically. Part of sharing the gospel with others is the substantiation of what sets us apart through Christ.

Self-control and endurance are easily authenticated by health and fitness. Discipline and diligence are easily demonstrated by a good diet and exercise. The difference is that we use the results to draw attention to God and live in a way that makes Jesus known. That is the goal of Christian faith inside and out. Peter puts it this way;

> *Therefore I intend always to remind you of these qualities . . . as long as I am in this body, to stir you up by way of reminder. . . . And I will make every effort so that after my departure you may be able at any time to recall these things.*

> —2 Pet. 1:12–13, 15

Peter knew we only get one life to do it right. We all get one chance to make an impact for the kingdom and leave something behind. So Peter made time for what he valued, for what he held dear. He devoted his body and mind exclusively to the message of the gospel. Faith-infused training helps us set aside time to strengthen the bodies God has given us. Take a moment to think about what time you could give up to better your health and get in better shape in light of what God has given up for you.

It might mean waking up before the sun comes up or getting to bed early. It might mean having a job where you're not working 50 to 60 hours a week or traveling all the time. For me, it was fasting from entertainment. The average American watches five hours and four minutes of television daily, while social media takes up nearly two hours of each person's day. Turning off the tube and shutting off my phone freed up at least 30 to 45 minutes for burning fat and building muscle. Pray and ask God what He might have you do differently.

Examine Your Heart

Think about this, too. What are your most common thoughts, your repeated deeds, and your regular actions? When what we say, think, and do are self-centered and self-focused, it reveals that either we aren't listening to God or we don't yet know how to listen to God. Ignoring the Holy Spirit who lives inside of us can be a very unhealthy thing. It's like living as if God doesn't exist. If our tendency is to wake up every morning to eat and drink whatever we want without being still and slowing down to consider the work of God, we could be in danger of laying down an infamous, weak foundation for ourselves.

You do not know what tomorrow will bring. What is your life? For you are a mist that appears for a little time and then vanishes. Instead you ought to say, "If the Lord wills, we will live and do this or that." As it is, you boast in your arrogance. All such boasting is evil. So whoever knows the right thing to do and fails to do it, for him it is sin.

—James 4:14–17

Part of building our bodies on the rock is submitting everything to the lordship of Jesus. It means finding our identity in Him so the master's touch is on us, our families, our relationships, our careers, our hobbies, and so on. We give everything over to Him because He gave His everything for us. Our plans, our schedule, and our money should all flow from a heart devoted to God. Search the scriptures and listen to Jesus's words. Along with showing us how to follow Him, He tells us the things we must surrender to God in radical faith.

What Do You Hold Dear?

Jesus says:

For where your treasure is, there your heart will be also.

—Matt. 6:21

What do our finances reveal about our hearts? When I took a look at my bank statements and credit card statements, a large portion of my money was being spent on food and drinks that damaged my body rather than improve it. It seemed like health and fitness were the last things I wanted to invest in. I was more concerned with building my body on what satisfied my cravings. During that time, Jesus may have been Lord over my spiritual issues, but salvation from anxiety and stress lay within a bowl of ice cream, a big fat plate of nachos, and a few shots of tequila.

There was a season in my life when I worked in multiple stressful environments. I was known more as a regular at the local bar than a regular at the local church. I literally lived off fast food, cigarettes, and energy drinks by day. My nights were spent freeing my mind with endless rounds of tall vodka tonics. Twenty-five bucks a day on junk and 25 bucks a night on booze added up to nearly $1,500 dollars per month. Here are a few things I've learned since then. Greasy foods and alcoholic beverages are among the worst culprits for hair loss and love handles, carbon monoxide doesn't increase stamina, caffeine begins with a high but ends in a crash, and hangovers and heart palpitations are no fun at all.

What I felt God was saying to me in the midst of all this was that if I didn't make a change, I was going to die. If I didn't redirect my finances toward sustenance and well-being, my lifestyle was going to destroy me. But God didn't want me to do it alone. He was going to be my ultimate source for recovery, the bedrock of my health, and the keystone of my strength. He did all this so He could win my heart and Christ could be my treasure.

Before any of us get fit, back in shape, or on the right track, we should fast and pray that God would reveal to us what we're currently building our body on. In order for God to be our firm foundation, we must create opportunities to listen further to the words of Jesus.

The Next Step: Stand and Walk

But seek first the kingdom of God and His righteousness, and all these things will be added to you.

—Matt. 6:33

Too many times, I've found myself focused on the wrong things. It was easy for me to get caught up in the "stuff" of life. Fine dining and fashionable wardrobes were what I sought after even with the knowledge that life is more than food and the body more than clothing (Luke 12:23). I never wanted to be waiting for God to provide. I wanted to be out there hustling, making money, contributing to my materialistic needs, and making a name for myself. That's what made me feel good.

I thought along the same lines with my body. It was easy to get caught up chasing rock-hard abs, a ripped physique, and a body that resembles a superman or an incredible hulk. I sold myself short trying to imitate the strength of super heroes, frankly because they don't exist. I avoided the living God whose strength is real and remains active. The strength of Christ, the solid rock, is real. He walked this earth until His death on a cross for us all, yet His power stays alive. He took a stance for us against pain and suffering, depression and hopelessness. It's time to stand and walk with Him.

Let's be super heroes of the faith like Moses. Let our legacy be in Christ with God.

> *Moses was 120 years old when he died. His eye was undimmed, and his vigor unabated. . . . And there has not arisen a prophet since in Israel like Moses, whom the Lord knew face to face, none like him for all the signs and the wonders that the Lord sent him to do.*
>
> —Deut. 34:7, 10–11

After Moses passed away, it was the prophet Joshua who stepped up to lead God's people. Joshua had spent his life training himself and others in the Lord to be fit for God's work. He was a warrior for Israel, a soldier in God's army. Since he had built his life on the rock and devoted his body in service to God's purpose, he was strengthened and protected by the supernatural power of the almighty.

Every place that the sole of your foot will tread upon I have given to
you, just as I promised.... No man shall be able to stand before you all
the days of your life.... I will be with you.... Only be strong and very
courageous, being careful to do according to all the law that Moses My
servant commanded you. Do not turn from it ... meditate on it day
and night.... For then you will make your way prosperous, and then
you will have good success.

—Josh. 1:3, 5, 7–8

The time came for Joshua to be in command, to spearhead a war with 40,000 men behind him and bring God's people to the Promised Land. But his legacy would not be dependent upon his own strength or by winning the battles. It would lie securely in the strength of God who would provide victory through His people's obedience to His word.

Follow Godly Examples

Standing and walking with Jesus means rising up and moving forward in the direction God leads us. It means paying attention to the details, being in tune with what God is speaking to our minds, our bodies, and our souls. For Joshua, that meant healthily leading God's people, setting the example for dedicating their bodies to a sacred purpose, and maintaining the strength and stamina to do so.

Traveling everywhere on foot wasn't easy, especially while carrying weighty objects such as the ark of the covenant, the tabernacle, their tents, food supplies, and all their gear for battle. Living for God isn't always lying down in green pastures. For Joshua, it meant tirelessly fighting the good fight, being fearlessly above reproach, and unashamedly serving God with boldness.

For us, rising up and moving forward might look a little different. It might mean simply getting up off the couch and being done with laziness. Or it could mean relocating to a foreign country where Christians are being persecuted for sharing the gospel. Whatever it looks like, we can be sure our minds and our souls need to be spiritually equipped for obedience and our bodies physically equipped for God's best.

How do we know what condition we're in? Who are the people around us in our circles who are building their bodies on the rock? If we need help to stand and walk, we should rally behind them for support. Then, once we've improved our bodies, we can share our testimony and be a support to others to be stronger and healthier. Having physical fitness mentors and being physically fit disciples will serve to strengthen our faith and our spiritual health.

Move Forward with Confidence

Posture is an important part of standing and walking, both physically and spiritually. It reveals what's going on with us inside and out. When I was completely out of shape, a good litmus test for me was knowing how quickly I would run out of breath. Instead of using elevators or escalators, I would take the stairs at a normal pace. I was surprised how little time it took before I started breathing heavily and my heart rate shot through the roof. I also noticed that while I worked, I had to sit down, lean on something, or slouch.

During that dark season of my life, I wasn't building my body on the rock, and other people knew it. I put on nearly 25 pounds of fat, which caused me to move more slowly and suffer from quite a bit of back pain. I was in a depressing trance most of the day, exhausted and drowsy. I wasn't seeking help from anyone, and I was too embarrassed to be seen in the gym.

My spiritual life was also plummeting. At church, I'd sit in random spots in the back rows, rarely participating in worship or communion. At the time, I was hardly obeying God in anything, so I felt guilty. It wasn't until God got me back on my feet, back on solid ground, that I was able to stand upright and walk in the strong, courageous way He commanded Joshua.

There were three evidences in the story of the Battle of Jericho that proved Joshua's spiritual posture enabled him to exercise physical poise for victory and success. The first was his preparatory submission. On the way to Jericho, he encountered the commander of God's army, Jesus. Immediately he responded in reverential awe, ready to do whatever it took to see God's promises fulfilled.

> *And Joshua fell on his face to the earth and worshiped and said to him, "What does my lord say to his servant?" And the commander of the LORD's army said to Joshua, "Take off your sandals from your feet, for the place where you are standing is holy." And Joshua did so.*
>
> —Josh. 5:14–15

The second evidence was Joshua's God-centered ambition. God gave Joshua specific instructions to win the battle, which he followed to a T. He led the priests and the armed soldiers through seven days of marching around the city walls, blowing trumpets continually, parading in full-dress uniform, with the ark of the covenant on display. None of the armed soldiers were allowed to take matters into their own hands nor were they allowed to even speak until the seventh day.

> *On the seventh day they rose early, at the dawn of day, and marched around the city in the same manner seven times. . . . And at the seventh time, when the priests had blown the trumpets, Joshua said to the people, "Shout for the LORD has given you the city. And the city and all that is in it shall be devoted to the LORD." . . . So the people shouted, and the trumpets were blown. . . . The people shouted a great shout, and the wall fell down flat . . . and they captured the city.*
>
> —Josh. 6:15–17, 20

The final confirmation was his unwavering passion. Without hesitation, Joshua did all that God required in high-caliber fashion. Carrying out such an unusual fight strategy with no questions asked said a lot about Joshua's patient leadership, his faith-infused action, and his strong desire to see God glorified. And the fact that God remained with Joshua through it all speaks highly of Joshua's genuine devotion to God's will. Joshua put his life in God's hands, creating an unbreakable bond, and should his legend grow, it would reflect the majesty of his king forever.

So the LORD was with Joshua, and his fame was in all the land.
—Josh. 6:27

The Last Step: Connect and Commit

Whether your quest is Olympic gold or a championship ring or a crown, building your body on the rock extends a humble invitation for God to participate in and maximize your glory and success. Whether you're a bodybuilder, a competitor, or a simple fitness nut, feeling good and looking good should always be pursued through God who sustains us and Christ who completes us. Whether your goal is to simply put on 20 pounds of muscle or take off 20 pounds of fat, let God tell you exactly what the game plan is. Pay attention to the details. Stick to His program for you no matter what, and let Him guide you into victory. Remember that health and fitness begin with God. So after you've fasted and prayed, after you stand and walk, and before you go run and lift, you must connect and commit. Make a heartfelt connection with other believers in your church or any church that has a hunger for the kind of strength that serves a higher purpose. Find out who's already treating their bodies as God's temple and join them. Make a wholehearted commitment to preparing for the physical work of God and to serving others by caring for your body, training yourself up in community.

The work of God is about people. The legacy of Joshua was never about the exaltation of one man. It was not a testimony about making it to the top, self-achievement, or never quitting. It's the story of one man who exalted God above all—above life and love, above money and fame, and above power and success. Joshua led God's people into their long-awaited inheritance. Let God use your body to minister to all people.

> *But as for me and my house, we will serve the LORD.*
> —Josh. 24:15

Working out religiously on your own is never enough. A significant part of building your life on the rock is being a blessing to others, sacrificing time and energy to meet spiritual and physical needs. Don't just think on personal levels when it comes to health and fitness. Think locally, nationally and globally.

Get to know your neighbors, your town, your city. Share your testimony of spiritual and physical fitness with everyone so when the time comes, you can provide them with strong hands and feet that are planted on solid ground. Get to know other Christians in your midst. They are your spiritual family. I guarantee you that there are believers who need your help and could also help you. None of us is as strong as all of us. And if all of us live in the strength of Christ, empowered by the Holy Spirit, there is no limit to what we can accomplish.

Conclusion

After hearing that I was writing *Faith-Infused Training*, a few people offered comments such as these: "Ya know, the moment you publish this book, your health and fitness will be under the microscope for as long as you live. Everyone will be paying close attention to what you eat and drink and to what your body looks like."

My response was that I wouldn't want it any other way. I need full transparency for full accountability. It was my lack of those things that ruined my health in the first place. I need to know, in all areas of my life, where I'm falling short, where I have issues, and where I'm being dominated by something other than the love of God. We, as God's people, need to be constantly aware of our tendency to choose death as a substitute for life, disease instead of health, and wrong over right.

So, under the microscope or not, we should always be transparent when it comes to what we're doing with our bodies. That way, while we live on mission for God, the light of our health and fitness can easily shine brightly into a dark, unhealthy world. We won't be perfect at it, but remember, we have the perfect example to follow. Just as Jesus, for the perfect joy that was set before Him, endured all things, we too, by His strength, can endure all things.

Right now, God is on mission everywhere, using His people around the world regardless of size, weight, condition, or shape. But when we join the battle against all hindrances, spiritually and physically, we maximize the effect and impact God has on us and others, all to attain a victory greater than we ever dreamed. When we join the fight to increase our bodily strength and elevate our mental focus, we become greater in Christ to achieve a higher level of growth that we never thought was possible. In doing so, we break through plateaus and biblically take everything up a notch, producing a faith-infused body of Christ that is relentless.

Our goal is to take the world by storm with ministry that spreads the all-encompassing love of God, to proclaim His good news with every inch of our bodies, and to protect His good name with every ounce of our souls—even if that means making drastic changes and going to extreme measures.

Long ago, I left the bar business because I got tired of feeding people junk food and getting them drunk night after night.

But while writing this book, I had to reconsider my career in the fast-food industry. Day after day, week after week, I was handing out greasy bags full of food that shouldn't be consumed as regularly as some do. Managing the drive-through was tough because customers would order fried sandwiches, fried vegetables, and over-sized sodas directly from me. Then I'd get a split second to glance in their cars and see empty wrappers and trash from other fast-food places, not to mention that a lot of them were obese, seemingly too out of shape to even get out of their car and walk into a restaurant to get their food.

I'm not judging anyone, but I was desperately wanting to see people's lives changed through a biblical perspective of health and fitness. So being in that atmosphere became too overwhelming. I reached a point where I felt as if I were perpetuating the cycle of obesity and excessive weight gain. Meanwhile, my own eating habits were changing for the good. God was doing a work in me through my experience in putting this book together. I had no other choice but to give my two weeks' notice and take a leap of faith to leave, knowing that God would provide for me and my family in my decision to follow His spirit elsewhere.

We mustn't ignore our convictions. And when it comes to our bodies, we mustn't ignore the red flags that the Holy Spirit will put up regarding improper diet, bad drinking habits, and the negative impact they can have on us spiritually and physically. Together, we must fight against all of it. But the journey will differ from person to person. That's why you didn't find any specific workout plans or diet programs in this book.

I stayed away from BMI graphs and fat percentage charts, because the issue isn't necessarily about the numbers. It's about your foundation, your attitude toward God. Remember, the heart of the issue is first spiritual and then physical. Without your heart, you can't live, but without the heart of Christ, you can't live forever. Having hearts, minds, souls, and bodies for Jesus is our endgame.

The end goal is to think and act like Christ—for our lives to look like His. That means lives filled with strength, courage, and commitment. Jesus is our model for how we think and act and how we steward our bodies. He will do His work in our hearts to guide us to wherever we need to go and whatever we need to do. If we end up with six-pack abs, great! But if not, we have something greater at our core: the living God.

Whether we struggle with being overweight or underweight, our bodies are God's temple. The Holy Spirit will always lead us in the charge to jettison sickness and infirmity so we can be thrust into biblically defined health and fitness. So let the condition of your heart and soul before God drive your training. Let your faith in Jesus be the deciding factor in why you diet and how you work out. As you take everything you want for your life and make it everything God wants for your life, you will hear Him say, loud and clear:

Well done, good and faithful servant. You have been faithful over a little; I will set you over much. Enter into the joy of your master.

—Matt. 25:23

I'm praying for you as you pray for me, to enter into the joy of God our master, physically and spiritually, now and forever. God bless.

Acknowledgments

It would be a crime not to mention the many people and organizations whose voices echo through the pages of this book and whose fingerprints are all over its words and content. Their support and prayers served as a driving force on every page and in every paragraph. Recognizing them here is both my way of showing gratitude for them and communicating what an honor and a privilege it is to know them.

First and foremost, to my wife, Brittany: Tears of love fill my eyes when I think about the sacrifices you made and everything you had to go through in order for God to bring us to where we are today. Thank you for putting up with me and for sleeping through the glowing screen of my computer and the sound of my fingers hitting the keyboard. I love you, and I promise, the best is yet to come.

To my kids: Michael and Nicholas, Trace and Dakota, and baby Ezra, I love you more than you know.

To all my family and friends everywhere: Every time I see you, I am thankful to God for another day of life and love.

To my pastors: Jason Shepperd, author of *Church Project: A Biblical, Simple, and Relevant Pursuit of Church*, thank you for all you do for the kingdom. Tierce Green, founder of Authentic Manhood Houston, love you, bro. Trace Howard, author of *Excellence in Planning and Promotion*, when I grow up, I want to be just like you. Hans Molegraaf, founder of Marriage Revolution, thank you for teaching me how to count my wife more significant than myself. George Booth, Jason Skaer, Rob Richie, John Shaw, Jonas Dienner, Calvin Taylor, and Airrion Fontenot, thank you for picking up your cross daily and being faithful men of the word of God.

To Josh and Ashley Lee for their ongoing support. To Eriek Hulseman for his guidance and honest feedback. To Angelia Griffin, author of *Just Winging It* and founder of AGF Publishing, for her wisdom and insight. To Jean Muñoz, my dear sister in Christ and devoted friend. To James Cook, president and founder of 12Two Missions. To Khari Gaynor, my FIT Brother in Christ and prayer warrior. To Erika Geier, founder and owner of Erika Geier Photography, thank you for taking the time to do my headshot. I'm also grateful for Aron and Stephanie Harris, Chris and Courtney Quinto, Dane and Paola Hall, Shawn and Serina Truhlar, Bill and Sandra Eaton, and Larry and Christi Till.

And to the church that meets at the Howorths' house: Thank you, my brothers and sisters, for everything.